Exploring and Teaching Healthcare Communication

Jack Pun

Exploring and Teaching Healthcare Communication

Clinicians' Perspectives in Hong Kong

palgrave
macmillan

Jack Pun
Department of English
The Chinese University of Hong Kong
Hong Kong SAR, China

ISBN 978-3-031-08674-8 ISBN 978-3-031-08675-5 (eBook)
https://doi.org/10.1007/978-3-031-08675-5

Cover credit: Thing Nong Nont | GettyImages

This Palgrave Macmillan imprint is published by the registered company Springer Nature Switzerland AG.
The registered company address is: Gewerbestrasse 11, 6330 Cham, Switzerland

This book is dedicated to patients, their families, and the healthcare professionals in Hong Kong who navigate the complexities of bilingual communication with empathy, expertise, and a deep respect for cultural diversity.

Acknowledgements

This book owes its existence to the collective efforts and steadfast support of numerous individuals and institutions who contributed to its creation. I am deeply grateful to the healthcare professionals, educators, and researchers whose invaluable insights and expertise have shaped my preparation for this book. Your dedication to enhancing healthcare communication in Hong Kong and beyond has been an enduring source of inspiration.

My heartfelt thanks go to the patients and families who courageously shared their experiences, challenges, and stories. Your voices underscore the critical role of compassionate, effective communication in healthcare, serving as a powerful reminder of its significance. Special recognition is extended to the interdisciplinary team of healthcare providers who provided lots of insights from their disciplines which have enriched this book with their diverse perspectives. I am also grateful for the thoughtful feedback and constructive suggestions from our colleagues and collaborators, which have significantly enhanced the content and depth of this book.

I wish to acknowledge the exceptional contributions of Ms Audrey Chan, whose invaluable support helped me to work on this book project. My sincere thanks also go to the reviewers whose insightful comments and suggestions have improved the quality of this work. Lastly, I express my deepest gratitude to the staff at Springer, particularly Mr Raghupathy

Kalyanaraman and Ms Cathy Scott, for their unwavering guidance and assistance throughout the process. To the readers of this book—healthcare practitioners, educators, policymakers, and students—this work is dedicated to you. I hope these pages serve as a meaningful resource to advance healthcare communication practices and foster greater understanding and collaboration across disciplines in bilingual context. Thank you all for being part of this journey to improve the teaching and learning of healthcare communication in Hong Kong.

Contents

About the Author

Jack Pun is an associate professor in the Department of English at the Chinese University of Hong Kong, Hong Kong SAR, China. He completed his PhD at the University of Oxford. As a bilingual speaker of Chinese and English, he is motivated to investigate the effectiveness and patient satisfaction of health communication from a cross-cultural and cross-disciplinary perspective. He explores the role of communication in shaping decision-making processes at consultations, and how communication affects the quality of care patients received from the health providers in different clinical settings (i.e. Emergency Department, Intensive Care Unit, Nursing Handovers, Traditional Chinese Medicine, Veterinary Medicine) and how effective communication enhances our understanding of the challenges and expectations in healthcare in worldwide hospital settings. *He is a founding member of the Institute for Communication in Healthcare (ICH) at the Australian National University, ANU, Canberra, Australia.* He is associate editor of the *Journal of Research in Science & Technological Education*, and published a recent monograph, *The Role of Language in Eastern and Western Health communication*, by Routledge.

1

Introduction

Researching and Teaching Healthcare Communication in Hong Kong: An Interdisciplinary and Intercultural Perspective

Healthcare in Hong Kong traverses a unique mix of Western and Chinese values, thus offering a comparative basis for evaluating cross-cultural expectations, practices, and experiences, consisting of elements of healthcare system from the East and the West. Particularly over the last decade, we have seen an interesting interest in exploring the role of clinical communication. In Asia, we witnessed a growing interest in implementing effective health communication and a trend of moving beyond a preference for Western-based communication practices by recognizing the local culture and expectations. The book urges the need to develop specific culturally appropriate communication models and provides recommendations from Chinese clinicians' perspective, which may ultimately improve therapeutic relationships and ensure patient safety.

This book brings together clinicians around patient care in different clinical contexts. This includes Medicine, Intensive care, Neurology,

J. Pun, *Exploring and Teaching Healthcare Communication*,
https://doi.org/10.1007/978-3-031-08675-5_1

Geriatrics, Oncology, Palliative care, Nursing, Clinical Psychology, Physiotherapy, Traditional Chinese Medicine and Veterinary Medicine. Drawing from these interprofessional approaches to communication, this book aims to provide evidence-based and practical suggestions to teach, research, and implement effective communication in Chinese contexts, addressing individual local cultural expectations. This book includes clinicians', and healthcare practitioners' up-to-date, frontline experiences, and their valuable advice on delivering and teaching effective clinical communication from Chinese perspectives. Each chapter begins with a summary of the nature of effective clinical communication in each discipline. It follows data emerged from the video-/audio-recorded expert interviews from a wide range of clinical contexts. These interview excerpts of up-to-date, practical experiences from the clinicians provide in-depth discussions and descriptions of the cultural difference between the healthcare system from the East and the West, with a focus on how Chinese Philosophy and cultural values underpin the effective clinical communication practice identified by these healthcare providers. It also describes how Chinese patients and healthcare practitioners precede themselves at clinical encounters at various stages of a patient journey. The book covers various topics on aspects of communication (i.e., stages of patient journeys, history taking, diagnosis, delivering bad news, treatment planning) and different elements of communication (i.e., Chinese culture, end-of-life communication, family role in communication) that are unique to Chinese contexts.

The chapters are informed by theory, research, and/or clinical practices, and will be of value to many clinical educators, allied health professionals, doctors/nurses in training, medical students; health communication researchers, students, and those already working or researching in the field. This book is particularly relevant to clinicians, healthcare providers, and medical educators from Chinese context, and also around the globe where non-Chinese clinicians need to communicate with Chinese patients and their carers.

International Teaching Tendency in East Asia: The Significance of Training Culturally Competent Medical Professionals

Over the past few decades, we have witnessed a growing research concern about communication problems that arise in intercultural contexts in East Asia. The nature of medical services are becoming more and more complicated in the stated settings because of the increasing emphasis on providing effective relational practices, implementing patient-centred care, ensuring patient safety, and the influences of cultural norms on healthcare discussions (Armah et al., 2020). As East Asian societies gradually turned into culturally diverse environments, practitioners, policymakers and medical professionals have learned that it is insufficient to directly apply the commonly used Calgary-Cambridge guides in English-speaking countries to their working spaces. Although researchers recognize the need for culturally sensitive communication models, only a minority have attempted to translate Westernized communication frameworks into culturally appropriate versions for Chinese healthcare providers and patients. As a result, researchers and seniors in hospitals should not neglect the significance of undergraduate medical training as well as post-qualification training programmes (Zou, 2016).

Intercultural clinical communication is a key to bridge clinicians and their patients across cultures in this globalized era. Only by then, different parties can meet their mutual treatment goals (Okech et al., 2015). The notion of intercultural communication covers elements from many cultural aspects, including gender dynamics, taboos, family relationships, and disciplines. It is important for clinicians to be well-versed and familiarized with their patients' cultural needs in order to provide them with equal opportunities regardless of their race (Keys, 2010). This book thus observes the trend and integrates knowledge from the fields of linguistics and cultural studies, and then recommends strategies for clinicians and their students to achieve a sufficient level of intercultural communicative competence (ICC) (Crawford et al., 2017; Harder, 2018; Henderson et al., 2016; Wros & Archer, 2010), which will train them for communication with a culturally diversified group of patients (Deardorff, 2015;

Ruppel & Brahms, 2014). This book uses the multicultural environment of Hong Kong as a case study and it is an integration of Western and Chinese cultural norms. The chapters evaluate cross-cultural patient expectations, medical practices, clinicians' experiences across disciplines, and the cultural elements that form the hybrid healthcare systems on a comparative basis.

Emphasizing the Human Factors of Medical Communication: What Does Patient-Centred Care Mean to Patients from Different Cultural and Language Backgrounds in Various Disciplines

The author of this book and his research team have been dedicated to enhancing multidisciplinary communication and collaboration between clinicians, which can improve clinician-patient and clinician-clinician relationships across cultures. One of the results was the *International Charter for Human Values in Healthcare*. It delineates core values, analyses the role effective communication plays in enforcing these values, and shows examples for other researchers, healthcare policymakers and medical professionals to translate these values into practice (Rider et al., 2014). Readers are recommended to refer to this charter as a teaching tool to facilitate medical professionals and students in their understanding of the crucial aspects of the human elements of care. For example, they should help implement the practice of compassionate, ethical, and safe relationship-centred patient experience (Rider et al., 2014).

Hospital management and clinicians should take up the responsibility of establishing well-developed values and communicating effectively in multiple scenarios in different disciplines. These include prevention and health maintenance, illness diagnoses, treatment plans and recovery (Kreps & Bonaguro, 2009; Simpson et al., 1991; Silverman et al., 2013; Rider & Keefer, 2006; Gracey et al., 2005; Rider, 2010, 2011; Miller & Schmidt, 1999; Slade et al., 2014). Accrediting institutions should train their employees to be competent in both humanistic and communication skills across cultures and evaluate their competency in these skills (Rider, 2010). According to recent research projects, effective communication can be achieved through the basis of core values. Good communication between clinical colleagues and their patients can help improve health outcomes, the quality of healthcare, and both patient and clinician satisfaction simultaneously (Rider, 2010; Branch et al., 2009; Finset, 2014; Sutcliffe et al., 2004). Given that such human aspects of healthcare have not been made central to clinical communication, the charter was designed to help clinicians identify and outline a framework for values that are important to relevant cultures and languages (Rider et al., 2014). Based on this charter, the following chapters aim to lead clinicians and training students to learn three interdependent kinds of communication strategies. These include (1) content skills (i.e., what one speaks); (2) process skills (i.e., what one communicates, e.g., structures conversations, asks questions, listens and responds, relates to patients and other relevant parties, relays messages using non-verbal skills and language, involves their patients when making shared decisions, etc.); (3) perceptual skills (i.e., what one thinks and feels, e.g., applies clinical reasoning and other thought processes and feelings as well as the way one deals with them, has and demonstrates the appropriate attitudes, biases, assumptions, intentions, values and capacities, including showing compassion, mindfulness, integrity, respect and so on). This book aims to help students and clinicians learn these skills and enhance their awareness in the human aspects of clinical communication across disciplines and cultures.

Cultural Clashes: So What Exactly Do Asian Patients Want from Their Care?

When reviewing previous studies and evaluating primary data obtained from original interviews, this book adopts compositional approaches to gain a holistic view of clinical communication in East Asia and Hong Kong (Pun et al., 2018). Although compositional approaches tend to result in rather static and restrictive views of cultures, they are still invaluable tools for the learning of cultural elements and comparisons between rituals, practices, and beliefs between multiple cultural groups in socio-cultural settings. We can then strive to understand how these aspects of healthcare communication reflect specific sets of cultural elements (Hofstede, 1997, 2001).

In order to highlight the unique characteristics of intercultural clinical communication in Hong Kong in the later chapters, the following sub-sections first introduce a more general overview of healthcare discussions in relevant Asian contexts. They draw on Ishikawa and Yamazaki (2005), Hofstede (1980), and Hall's (1959) theoretical frameworks regarding the cultural collisions between Western clinical communication models and Asia-specific cultural norms (Pun et al., 2018). These sections focus on the tensions between individualism and collectivism; high-context and low-context cultures; gender dynamics; and Christian and Confucian values.

The Key Role of Families in Decision-Making Processes: The Hindering of Patient Autonomy

As per Ishikawa and Yamazaki (2005), Asian people tend to adhere to collectivist behaviours. This means that clinicians and patients' relatives often see the patients as a component of a bigger social unit. Contrarily, their Western counterparts emphasize patient autonomy and individual rights. This is particularly true when it comes to a patient's right to make their own End-Of-Life (EOL) decisions such as refusing any cardiopulmonary resuscitation after cardiac arrest. It is widely believed that clinicians' respect for patients' individual choices can successfully promote advance directives and improve the quality of EOL care (Eliott & Olver, 2007). On the other hand, Asian patients are seen as tightly bonded in-group members (Hofstede, 2001) who interdepend on their families when making decisions (Zhu, 2014). As a result, many clinicians often seek the relatives' opinions instead of just the patients themselves when making treatment plans (Back & Huak, 2005). However, recent studies have demonstrated that Asian patients, including those from Taiwan, have voiced their concerns about their individual rights when making decisions, especially regarding EOL matters. For instance, we have seen the percentages of

DNR orders (Do Not Resuscitate) and hospice care utilisation rocketing between 2008 and 2014 (Shih et al., 2017). Thus, clinicians based in Asia need to be culturally trained to learn the varying desired levels of patient autonomy across regions and be able to assess individual patient's unique circumstances in accordance with their cultural values.

Reading Non-verbal Cues in High-Context Cultures: Asia as the Feminine East

In high-context cultures, communication tends to be less explicit when compared to low-context ones in Europe and America. Zhu (2014) stated that low-context cultures including the United States and Mexico focus on the notions of heroism, achievement, determination as well as material success. Thus, important information is usually directly conveyed in communication. On the other hand, Japan, South Korea, and China are categorized as "feminine" high-context cultures that stress the importance of harmonious relations, hierarchy, humility, and care for the weak by Hofstede (2001). Therefore, many studies found that Asian patients would rather express their opinions and feelings implicitly through language or even non-verbal cues (Ohtaki et al., 2003). Therefore, clinicians need to learn to observe and tend to their patients' unspoken psycho-emotional needs.

The Confucian System of Societal Hierarchy: Clinicians and Patients

The different cultural norms and values form the nature of clinical communication in varying cultures (Scollon, 2000). This explains the variation between the features of Western and Eastern clinician-patient dynamics (Jin & Cortazzi, 1998). In Anglophone medical settings, both practitioners and patients pay attention to their interpersonal relationships and the implementation of patient-oriented care because of Christian beliefs. Parties in Asian regions wish to uphold harmony, show obedience to the authorial stakeholder, and show respect to seniors under

Confucian influences. Such Confucian beliefs result in hierarchical, paternalistic as well as asymmetrical clinician-patient dynamics (Ishikawa & Yamazaki, 2005).

That being said, Claramita et al.'s (2013) well-elaborated interviews with 20 clinicians and 20 patients showed that many patients were dissatisfied with their practitioners' one-way communication style. Hong Kong, for example, is a hybrid between the West and the East. This makes the patients shift to more Westernized thought processes. It is important to take that into consideration and read into context-specific variables including the social distance between clinicians and their patients, and thus tailor communication styles to each patient.

Identifying the Uniqueness of Each Culture: The Necessity to Carry Out Multicultural and Interdisciplinary Case Studies

Although it is useful and convenient for researchers to generalize cultural differences between Asian and Western communication, such attribution can lead to cultural essentialism (Zhu, 2014). It is important for researchers and clinicians to not stereotype their patients based on cultural assumptions. Therefore, this book uses Hong Kong as a case study to learn how Western and Chinese medical communication features and values blend with each other. The diverse nature of Hong Kong enables researchers to assess the emergence of cross-cultural patient expectations, real-life practices, and experiences. The following chapters offer guidance for clinicians to adopt culturally appropriate communication strategies according to their patients' cultural exposure to Western and Traditional Chinese Medicine. The case of Hong Kong can be read as a reflection of the increasingly globalized scene of medical services in general. Thus, researchers and medical professionals across the world can refer to these case studies when forming multicultural and multilingual frameworks for clinical communication.

Chapter Synopsis

Chapter 1: Introduction

This current chapter is an introduction to the topic of this book. It describes the background of exploring, researching, and teaching effective clinical communication in general. It also offers a brief overview of previous research and research findings from the healthcare system between the East and the West. It further provides an outline of the subsequent chapters of the book and highlights the significance of the research.

Chapter 2: Researching Communication in Chinese Contexts

Chapter 2 examines previous studies on clinical communication in Asia, highlighting priorities that emerged from Chinese research, such as family orientation, Chinese philosophical foundations for effective communication, and the concept of a good death. This chapter critically assesses these priorities using research evidence from existing literature to illustrate their manifestation in the Chinese context. Additionally, it maps key theories and practices from both Chinese and non-Chinese contexts, creating a narrative that demonstrates how the current project diverges from and contributes to the field, extending existing theories or frameworks.

Chapter 3: Understanding Communication in Critical Care: Clinicians' and Patients' Perspectives

This chapter investigates the complexities of clinical communication in two critical care settings in Hong Kong: the Intensive Care Unit (ICU) and the Accident & Emergency Department (AED). It examines the multilingual challenges posed by the use of Cantonese, Mandarin, and

English in clinician-patient and inter-clinician interactions, focusing on their impact on patient care quality, safety, and outcomes.

Drawing on interviews with ICU and AED clinicians, the chapter explores recurring themes in communication practices, including the dynamics of shared decision-making, the barriers to effective collaboration, and the unique linguistic challenges of trilingual environments. It further incorporates perspectives from mechanically ventilated (MV) patients in ICUs, shedding light on their unmet communication needs and the psycho-emotional impacts of limited verbal interaction.

Findings reveal significant obstacles, such as hierarchical dynamics, time constraints, limited resources, and inconsistent documentation practices. In the ICU, the chapter emphasizes the importance of fostering a "speak-up" culture to empower clinicians to voice concerns and improve interdisciplinary collaboration. In the AED, it highlights the risks of code-switching, translation errors, and the pressure of high patient volumes, which compromise the clarity of medical documentation and patient understanding.

The chapter concludes by proposing practical frameworks to enhance communication effectiveness in high-stress, multilingual medical environments. These include strategies to promote patient-centred communication, align interdisciplinary goals, and address systemic barriers to clear and empathetic interactions in ICUs and AEDs. The recommendations offer a roadmap for improving healthcare delivery and patient safety in Hong Kong's critical care contexts.

Chapter 4: Researching Clinician-to-Clinician Communication at Handovers

This chapter examines clinician-to-clinician communication during nursing handovers in Hong Kong hospitals, emphasizing the complexities of transitions in care within multilingual and multicultural healthcare settings. Using an ethnographic discourse analysis approach, the study explores handover practices in medical and surgical wards, drawing on recorded handover sessions and interviews with hospital administrators, nurse managers, and frontline nursing staff. The research highlights the structural and interactional patterns of handovers, shedding light on how clinicians convey critical patient information and navigate communication challenges.

Key findings reveal the need for improving handover practices through systematic and evidence-based strategies. These include:

1. Adopting a structured framework for presenting information to ensure clarity and reduce risks.
2. Promoting active engagement from incoming nurses by encouraging verification and clarification of details.
3. Ensuring explicit responsibility transfer by outgoing nurses through confirmation and readback protocols.
4. Integrating verbal handovers with access to written documentation to support comprehensive communication.

The study underscores the impact of multilingual and hierarchical dynamics on handover communication, examining the effectiveness of the ISBAR protocol in this context. It also introduces the CARE model, designed to enhance collaborative and patient-centred interactions during handovers, fostering a culture of active participation and mutual understanding.

By analysing communication at both macro and micro levels, this chapter contributes to the broader understanding of clinician-to-clinician interactions in high-pressure environments. It provides actionable recommendations for improving handover communication, aligning with global efforts to advance patient safety, care quality, and professional development in healthcare settings.

Chapter 5: Understanding High-Risk Multilingual Communication in Accident & Emergency Departments (AED)

This chapter examines the nature of doctor-patient communication in one of the AEDs in Hong Kong. It sums up the complexity of communication in the trilingual context of clinical communication in the city and shows language evidence of patient participation in shared decision-making processes during AED visits. The chapter includes results from interviews with key AED clinicians on their experience regarding the patient journey from triage to disposition. It thematically analyses the data to highlight the recurring factors in clinicians' communication practices, which forms the basis for the investigation of the linguistic evidence of shared patient decision-making processes and the communication challenges that emerge in trilingual interactions.

The findings demonstrate the major barriers that hinder effective communication that arise from the use of spoken Chinese (including both Cantonese and Mandarin) during doctor-patient consultations, code-mixing between Chinese and English in clinician-clinician communication and the use of written English in medical documentation. This chapter investigates how such an immense level of communicative complexity influences the quality of patient journeys and the accuracy of information relay. The chapter also discusses other challenges to patient safety and the experience in the AED, including the lack of information that informs the processes of running an AED, time pressure and the constant lack of manpower, differences in goals between doctors and patients, how diagnoses and treatment plans are delivered inefficient and the consequent absence of patient compliance, and how hierarchy brings negative impacts on care. The chapter concludes by offering a model for future researchers in Hong Kong to improve the effectiveness of healthcare communication from a multilingual perspective.

Chapter 6: Chinese Clinicians' Perspectives Towards Inter- and Intra-disciplinary Communication Between Staff in the Intensive Care Unit

This chapter details observations of the speak-up culture within an ICU at a hospital in Hong Kong. The findings show doctors' and nurses' perceptions of communication openness during both intra- and interdisciplinary interactions. The reported study measured the quality of ICU teamwork through a validated cross-sectional survey. The chapter discusses insights from 80 ICU staff towards their views on speak-up culture and their self-reported ability to have open conversations. Ten individuals who showed high communication openness in the survey were asked to participate in an audio-recorded observation of their clinical practices. Semi-structured interviews were then carried out for researchers to identify factors that impacted the speak-up culture in the said ICU, the critical moments for speaking up, and their motivations for engaging in effective speak-up practices. The chapter concludes with suggestions for clinicians and hospital management to foster a secure environment and emphasize the importance of equal status. These strategies aim to help team members feel confident in communicating openly and sharing their personal opinions without fear of retaliation or embarrassment.

Chapter 7: Teaching Clinical Communication to Medical Students in Hong Kong

Teaching clinical communication in Hong Kong's medical education system presents unique challenges due to the intersection of Western medical frameworks and Chinese cultural expectations. Existing models such as SPIKES and the Calgary-Cambridge guide, while widely used, often fail to address the local sociocultural and linguistic needs, particularly when students must communicate in first language (i.e., Cantonese) and engage with family members in decision-making. In this bilingual environment, such as Hong Kong, clinicians frequently switch between conversational Cantonese (spoken) and technical medical English (written), navigating the complexities of balancing everyday language with medical terminology to effectively communicate with patients and provide culturally sensitive care. This chapter examines some current practices around teaching clinical communication and proposes a hybrid communication framework which perhaps can integrate Western models with culturally specific adaptations. The chapter also highlights the need for targeted training in local language use, culturally appropriate expressions of empathy, and navigating family dynamics. The chapter also advocates for a culturally informed approach to medical education in Hong Kong and calls for further research to assess the effectiveness of these proposed teaching practices in real-world practice.

Chapter 8: Educating Medical Students in Hong Kong on Clinical Communication: Emphasizing End-of-Life Conversations

Effective clinical communication is essential for medical students in Hong Kong, especially when addressing sensitive topics like end-of-life (EOL) care. This chapter explores the unique challenges of teaching EOL communication within Hong Kong's culturally diverse healthcare setting, where Western medical practices intersect with traditional Chinese values. In this context, family involvement, cultural norms surrounding death, and the balance between patient autonomy and familial decision-making play crucial roles in shaping EOL conversations. The chapter discusses the limitations of applying Western communication models, such as the SPIKES protocol, in Chinese settings and advocates for a culturally appropriate, hybrid model that incorporates both Western techniques and Chinese communication practices. Key teaching strategies include the use of simulated patient encounters, role-playing with real-life cases, and interdisciplinary collaboration to prepare students for complex clinical interactions. By fostering a deeper understanding of the cultural dimensions of communication, medical educators can equip students with the skills necessary to navigate EOL discussions effectively and compassionately, improving patient care in Hong Kong.

Chapter 9: Navigating Communication in Traditional Chinese Medicine: Strategies, Challenges, and Pedagogical Approaches

This chapter explores the distinctive communication strategies and challenges present within Traditional Chinese Medicine (TCM) consultations in Hong Kong. The chapter emphasizes TCM's holistic approach, which seeks to balance body, mind, and spirit, contrasting with the symptom-focused methodology of Western Medicine (WM). Drawing from recent studies on doctor-patient interactions, the chapter analyses the linguistic and discoursal techniques used by TCM practitioners, including structured questioning routines, discourse markers, and personalized inquiries into patients' daily lives. These strategies help establish trust, facilitate shared decision-making, and enhance patient participation. The chapter also examines the implications for TCM communication education, advocating for a tailored approach that incorporates patient-centred care principles while honouring the cultural dimensions unique to TCM practice. By offering practical strategies for educators and healthcare professionals, the chapter aims to enhance communication skills within TCM, thereby improving patient satisfaction and health outcomes. It further discusses the integration of WM communication models, demonstrating that the adoption of patient-centred techniques, such as those from the Calgary-Cambridge model, can strengthen rapport and increase patient satisfaction. The chapter concludes by stressing the importance of incorporating culturally relevant elements into TCM communication training, such as the development of long-term relationships and addressing interpersonal concerns, to elevate overall healthcare delivery in Hong Kong.

Chapter 10: Exploring Veterinary Medicine Communication in Hong Kong

This chapter delves into the essential role of communication in veterinary practice within Hong Kong's unique bilingual and multicultural environment. It examines the specific communication competencies needed by veterinary students to manage clinical interactions, including explaining diagnoses, discussing treatment plans, and documenting cases in professional formats. The chapter identifies key challenges posed by language barriers and cultural expectations, particularly in using English for professional purposes alongside Cantonese in client interactions. Emphasizing a client-centred and cross-disciplinary approach, the chapter advocates for a practical, multimodal curriculum that includes bilingual communication training and exercises in empathy, active listening, and teamwork. Drawing on research findings and practitioner insights, this chapter proposes innovative teaching methods to address the gap between academic instruction and clinical practice, aiming to better equip students for Hong Kong's diverse veterinary sector and enhance their readiness to meet both linguistic and professional standards.

Chapter 11: Conclusion

This chapter concludes the book by synthesizing key themes on clinical communication in Hong Kong context, particularly emphasizing the importance of culturally responsive communication strategies. With the coexistence of Western and Chinese medical practices, clinicians in Hong Kong must navigate cultural values like family-centred decision-making, high-context communication styles, and a holistic approach inherent to Traditional Chinese Medicine (TCM). These insights inform ethical challenges specific to clinical communication research in the region, such as obtaining informed consent within family-influenced contexts, managing video/audio recordings respectfully, and maintaining confidentiality. This chapter advocates a culturally integrated communication model that adapts Western approaches to align with the high-context, family-oriented nature of Chinese culture, promoting patient-centred care that respects both autonomy and cultural traditions. Towards the end, the author addresses ethical considerations in researching healthcare communication within Chinese contexts and explains the standard procedures for conducting such studies in Hong Kong.

Summary

To conclude, this chapter introduces healthcare communication in Hong Kong, emphasizing its unique integration of Western and Chinese cultural values. It traces the evolution of clinical communication in Asia, highlighting a gradual shift from predominantly Western frameworks to culturally tailored approaches that align with local traditions and societal expectations. The discussion underscores the importance of developing communication models that are both culturally appropriate and sensitive to the needs of Chinese patients and healthcare providers. These frameworks have the potential to foster stronger therapeutic relationships and enhance patient safety.

Hong Kong's healthcare system exemplifies a hybrid model, seamlessly blending Western medicine with Traditional Chinese Medicine (TCM). This integration not only showcases the possibilities for effective cross-cultural communication but also serves as a practical example of how healthcare systems can adapt to diverse cultural contexts. The chapter incorporates interdisciplinary perspectives by drawing on insights from various fields, including medicine, nursing, psychology, TCM, and even veterinary medicine, to provide a comprehensive understanding of effective healthcare communication strategies.

A significant focus of the chapter is on culturally informed communication, exploring how Chinese cultural values shape clinical interactions. These values include the emphasis on family involvement in medical decision-making, respect for end-of-life traditions, and reliance on high-context communication styles. Through clinician interviews and real-world examples, the chapter illustrates how these cultural elements influence the dynamics of healthcare interactions in Hong Kong.

The chapter also offers practical recommendations for teaching and researching healthcare communication. It highlights the importance of incorporating tools such as the *International Charter for Human Values in Healthcare*, which emphasizes the humanistic aspects of medical care. These suggestions aim to provide valuable insights for clinicians, medical educators, and students, facilitating the development of culturally competent healthcare practices.

In closing, the chapter advocates for fostering intercultural communicative competence (ICC) among healthcare professionals. It emphasizes the need for training programmes that integrate linguistic, cultural, and relational aspects of communication, enabling medical professionals to navigate Hong Kong's multicultural healthcare landscape effectively. By using Hong Kong as a case study, the chapter sets the stage for further exploration of hybrid healthcare systems, offering valuable insights for global applications.

References

Armah, N., Martin, D., Harder, N., & Deer, F. (2020). Undergraduate nursing students' perspectives of intercultural communication: A qualitative descriptive study. *Nurse Education Today, 95*, 104604.

Back, M. F., & Huak, C. Y. (2005). Family centred decision making and non-disclosure of diagnosis in a South East Asian oncology practice. *Psychooncology, 14*(12), 1052–1059.

Branch, W. T., Frankel, R., Gracey, C. F., et al. (2009). A good clinician and a caring person: Longitudinal faculty development and the enhancement of the human dimensions of care. *Academic Medicine, 84*, 117–125.

Claramita, M., Nugraheni, M. D., van Dalen, J., & van der Vleuten, C. (2013). Doctor–patient communication in Southeast Asia: A different culture? *Advances in Health Sciences Education, 18*(1), 15–31.

Crawford, T., Candlin, S., & Roger, P. (2017). New perspectives on understanding cultural diversity in nurse-patient communication. *Collegian, 24*(1), 63–69.

Deardorff, D. (2015). Intercultural competence: Mapping the future research agenda. *International Journal of Intercultural Relations, 48*, 3–5.

Eliott, J., & Olver, I. (2007). Autonomy and the family as (in) appropriate surrogates for DNR decisions: A qualitative analysis of dying cancer patients' talk. *The Journal of Clinical Ethics, 18*(3), 206–218.

Finset, A. (2014). 50 years of research on the effect of physician communication behavior on health outcomes. *Patient Education and Counseling, 96*, 1–2.

Gracey, C. F., Haidet, P., Branch, W. T., et al. (2005). Precepting humanism: Strategies for fostering the human dimensions of care in ambulatory settings. *Academic Medicine, 80*, 21–28.

Hall, E. T. (1959). *The Silent Language* (Vol. 3). Doubleday.

Harder, N. (2018). Determining the effects of simulation on intercultural competency in undergraduate nursing students. *Nurse Educator, 43*(1), 4–6.

Henderson, S., Barker, M., & Mak, A. (2016). Strategies used by nurses, academics and students to overcome intercultural communication challenges. *Nurse Educator, 16*(1), 71–78.

Hofstede, G. (1980). Culture and organizations. *International Studies of Management and Organization, 10*(4), 15–41.

Hofstede, G. (1997). Organization culture. In A. Sorge & M. Warner (Eds.), *The IBM Handbook of Organizational Behavior* (pp. 193–210). International Thomson Business Press.

Hofstede, G. (2001). *Culture's Consequences: Comparing Values, Behaviors, Institutions and Organizations Across Nations*. Sage Publications.

Ishikawa, H., & Yamazaki, Y. (2005). How applicable are western models of patient-physician relationship in Asia? Changing patient-physician relationship in contemporary Japan. *International Journal of Japanese Sociology, 14*(1), 84–93.

Jin, L., & Cortazzi, M. (1998). The culture the learner brings: A bridge or a barrier? In M. Byram & M. Fleming (Eds.), *Language Learning in Intercultural Perspectives: Approaches through Drama and Ethnography* (pp. 98–118). Cambridge University Press.

Keys, T. R. (2010). Behaviors that eliminate health disparities for racial and ethnic minorities: A narrative system. *Proceedings of the New York State Communication Association*, 1–24.

Kreps, G., & Bonaguro, E. (2009). Health communication as applied communication inquiry. In L. Frey & K. Cissna (Eds.), *Handbook of Applied Communication Research* (pp. 380–404). Routledge.

Miller, S. Z., & Schmidt, H. J. (1999). The habit of humanism: A framework for making humanistic care a reflexive clinical skill. *Academic Medicine, 74*, 800–803.

Ohtaki, S., Ohtaki, T., & Fetters, M. D. (2003). Doctor–patient communication: A comparison of the USA and Japan. *Family Practice, 20*(3), 276–282.

Okech, M., Asher, M., Pimpleton, R. V., & Julia, C. (2015). Intercultural communication: An application to group work. *The Journal for Specialists in Group Work, 40*(30), 268–293.

Pun, J., Chan, A. E., Wang, S., & Slade, D. (2018). Health professional-patient communication practices in East Asia: An integrative review of an emerging field of research and practice in Hong Kong, South Korea, Japan, Taiwan, and Mainland China. *Patient Education and Counseling, 101*(7), 1193–1206.

Rider, E. A. (2010). Interpersonal and communication skills. In E. A. Rider & R. H. A. Nawotniak (Eds.), *Practical Guide to Teaching and Assessing the ACGME Core Competencies* (pp. 1–173). HCProMarblehead.

Rider, E. A. (2011). Advanced communication strategies for relationship-centered care. *Pediatric Annals, 40*, 447–453.

Rider, E. A., & Keefer, C. H. (2006). Communication skills competencies: Definitions and a teaching toolbox. *Medical Education, 40*, 624–629.

Rider, E. A., Kurtz, S., Slade, D., et al. (2014). The International Charter for Human Values in Healthcare: An interprofessional global collaboration to

enhance values and communication in healthcare. *Patient Education and Counseling, 96*(3), 273–280.
Ruppel, P. S., & Brahms, K. S. (2014). Intercultural communication: Overview. In *Encyclopaedia of Critical Psychology* (pp. 970–974).
Scollon, S. (2000). Not to waste words or students: Confucian and Socratic discourse in the tertiary classroom. In E. Hinkel (Ed.), *Culture in Second Language Teaching and Learning* (pp. 13–27). Cambridge University Press.
Shih, T. C., Chang, H. T., Lin, M. H., Chen, C. K., Chen, T. J., & Hwang, S. J. (2017). Trends of do-not-resuscitate orders, hospice care utilization, and late referral to hospice care among cancer decedents in a tertiary hospital in Taiwan between 2008 and 2014: A hospital-based observational study. *Journal of Palliative Medicine, 20*(8), 838–844.
Silverman, J., Kurtz, S., & Draper, J. (2013). *Skills for Communicating with Patients*. Radcliffe Publishing.
Simpson, M., Buckman, R., Stewart, M., Maguire, C. P., Lipkin, M., Novack, D., & Till, J. (1991). Doctor–patient communication: The Toronto Consensus Statement. *British Medical Journal, 202*, 1384–1387.
Slade, D., Manidis, M., McGregor, J., et al. (2014). *Communicating in Hospital Emergency Departments*. Springer.
Sutcliffe, K. M., Lewton, E., & Rosenthal, M. (2004). Communication failures: An insidious contributor to medical mishaps. *Academic Medicine, 79*, 186–194.
Wros, P., & Archer, S. (2010). Comparing learning outcomes of international and local community partnerships for undergraduate nursing students. *Journal of Community Health Nursing, 27*(4), 216–225.
Zhu, H. (2014). *Exploring Intercultural Communication: Language in Action*. Routledge.
Zou, P. (2016). Relational practice in nursing: A case analysis. *Nursing & Health Care, 1*(1), 1–5.

2

Researching Clinical Communication in Chinese Contexts

The Implications of Interdisciplinary Applied Linguistics to Healthcare Communication Research

As introduced in the previous chapter, a key goal of this book is to investigate the ways in which healthcare workers work in multilingual Asian contexts and Chinese societies like Hong Kong from an interdisciplinary lens. This chapter elaborates on the interdisciplinary and ethnographic approaches used throughout the book under the scope of applied linguistics. It then reviews some of the overarching themes that emerged from previous interdisciplinary studies on healthcare communication in Asia and Hong Kong in particular. These introductory accounts of identified methodologies and key themes will give the reader an overview of research trends in healthcare communication in Asian contexts.

So what does interdisciplinary research mean in the area of applied linguistics? According to Stern, Stern, Taron, Stern, and Yule in *Fundamental Concepts of Language Teaching: Historical and Interdisciplinary Perspectives on Applied Linguistic Research* (1983), the concept of

J. Pun, *Exploring and Teaching Healthcare Communication*,
https://doi.org/10.1007/978-3-031-08675-5_2

"interdisciplinary" entails the following in relation to fundamental concepts and language teaching:

> language teaching research has certain specific characteristics which make it different from other educational research because its subject matter is language. Hence the research procedures of the language sciences are applicable. It is this *interdisciplinary combination of language research with educational and behavioural research* that gives language teaching research its unique characteristics and peculiar difficulties.
> (Stern et al., 1983, p. 63, italics my own)

Interdisciplinary studies in the area of applied linguistics emphasize the pedagogical implications of the approaches to the use of language and learning. The learning is achieved by the integration of knowledge from different fields, including linguistics, behavioural science, and education. Interdisciplinary healthcare communication studies have been widely conducted as the delivery of medical services is composed of exchanges and decisions mediated by cognitive, cultural, and sociolinguistic models or schemata (Cicourel, 1999). The goal of interdisciplinary projects is not to isolate a certain group and make assumptions about a practice being effective or ineffective for the entire group. Instead, these projects strive to make descriptive accounts of the event and its impact and evaluate the types of effects the practices have on the group (Roberts & Sarangi, 1999). For instance, it is crucial for clinicians, policymakers, and researchers to assess if the Western patient-centred healthcare philosophies are applicable to the role, context as well as emotion schemas in Chinese settings (Zhu, 2014). This is due to the major sociocultural differences between Western and Chinese contexts as culture is fundamentally a repository of attitudes and hierarchies (Samovar et al., 1998). The variations lead to different frameworks of medical care delivery and communication. Thus, it is essential for researchers to develop context-specific medical communication models. Interdisciplinary research designs can facilitate researchers in developing culturally appropriate healthcare communication models in multicultural contexts by emphasizing the influences of local cultural elements.

Defining "Interdisciplinary" Healthcare Communication Research

Decades ago, most researchers adopted disciplinarity research to their studies in the field of applied linguistics. In the contemporary world, issues have become more and more complex, and thus, there is a call for readings from multiple perspectives of different disciplines. By merging insights from various fields, researchers can engage in several steps to gain a holistic understanding of different situations. These steps include (1) utilizing existing knowledge from specific fields while consistently transcending it by integrating insights, (2) producing new knowledge through the research process while incorporating methods from a particular field when necessary, and (3) identifying research gaps and addressing them through interdisciplinary integration, which is often lacking in single-discipline studies (Repko et al., 2016). In short, interdisciplinary research is

> a process of answering a question, solving a problem, or addressing a topic that is too broad or complex to be dealt with adequately by a single discipline, and draws on the disciplines with the goal of integrating their insights to construct a more comprehensive understanding.
> (Repko et al., 2016, p. 15)

By concentrating deeply on intricate modern challenges that disciplinary research alone cannot fully address, interdisciplinary studies can generate pragmatic results that lead to new and comprehensive understandings (Bracken & Oughton, 2006; Klein, 2008; Lattuca, 2001; Metzger & Zare, 1999; Porter et al., 2006; Rhoten, 2004; Van Noorden, 2015; Varey, 1995). For instance, Brookes and Hunt's book *Analysing Health Communication Discourse Approaches* (2021) employs an interdisciplinary method by merging discourse analysis with studies in clinical communication. This integration allows researchers to drive initiatives, shape health behaviours, and advocate for significant transformations in both social and healthcare environments (Brookes & Hunt, 2021). Given the intricate nature of current global healthcare communication challenges, interdisciplinary approaches provide researchers with valuable tools to tackle the unique clinical communication issues found across various cultural settings.

An Overview of Themes in Chinese-Context Health Communication Studies: Interdisciplinary and Ethnographic Perspectives

This session integrates the interdisciplinary literature review conducted by Pun et al. (2018) and Pun et al. (2019) and offers an overview of some overarching themes in healthcare communication studies in Asian and Chinese contexts. Pun et al.'s (2018) review article identified and integrated research findings from numerous disciplinary studies, which offered us a glimpse into a set of recurring broad mutual themes in the studies of healthcare communication in East Asia. The article illustrated two key broad areas of themes, namely (1) parties that contribute to the formation of clinician-patient relationships, which consists of the involved parties' understanding of the roles and expectations of doctors, nurses, patients and their relatives; and (2) factors that impact that quality of medical care. Pun et al. (2019) adopted a socially oriented functional approach from the area of ethnography to integrate conflicting disciplinary ideas and their primary observations. The approach in turn allowed the researchers to learn about the ways nurses use languages in authentic, everyday clinical scenarios during communication with their patients and peers. The discussion of the following themes functions as an introductory guide to the major hindrances clinicians face when communicating for work in Hong Kong and other Asian and context contexts. The subsequent chapters will then further give directions to the development of culturally appropriate training courses for both pre- and post-qualification clinicians, and teach students in applied linguistics to carry out interdisciplinary health communication studies in Hong Kong.

What Are the Roles and Expectations of Clinicians, Patients, and Relatives in East Asia?

Emotional or Physical Comfort from Nurses?

In the broader East Asian context, understanding the roles and expectations of medical professionals, patients, and their families involves examining subthemes like nurse-patient communication, doctor-patient communication, and the role of family members. The review article synthesizes studies that highlight cultural distinctions between nurse-patient relationships in East Asia and the West within their respective medical systems. Interdisciplinary research shows that East Asian patients tend to value physical comfort provided by nurses over emotional support. This insight aligns with Jiang et al.'s (2015) research on the caring behaviours of 260 nurses in Shanghai, China (Jiang et al., 2015). Their findings suggest that nurses excel at providing technical care, such as using specialized equipment and administering treatments, but find it more difficult to express empathy and build rapport. Pun et al. (2018) contrasted these findings with Dong et al.'s (2016) study on terminal cancer patients in China, which revealed that nurses focused on physical comfort while doctors addressed symptoms and patients' rights (Dong et al., 2016). Liu et al. (2006) noted that the Chinese medical setting differs from Western ones due to cultural norms that treat bad news as a private, family matter, limiting nurses' involvement in difficult conversations. Furthermore, considering the cultural taboo surrounding death in China, the research team drew on cultural studies to recommend re-evaluating nurses' communication strategies with cancer patients in Chinese contexts (Pun et al., 2018).

Asymmetrical Dynamics Between Doctors and Patients

The reviewed literature revealed that doctor-patient relationships in East Asian contexts tend to be unequal (Ishikawa & Yamazaki, 2005). As Wang (2010) pointed out, patients in China generally prefer doctors to assume a more dominant role in communication, unlike patients in the United States. This preference, however, results in a doctor-centred communication model, leading to patient dissatisfaction, as they often face long waiting times for very brief consultations (Yin et al., 2012). Yin et al. also noted similar circumstances in Taiwan by analysing interactions between 6 senior paediatricians and their 30 patients, along with the patients' families (Yin et al., 2012).

This cultural aspect negatively affects patients' experiences. Siu's (2015) study on communication between female patients with overactive bladders and male urologists in Hong Kong found that patients often felt embarrassed and had limited options regarding their treatment plans. Hsiao et al. (2006) explained that traditional gender roles in Chinese culture make male doctors less empathetic, as patriarchal norms discourage men from being expressive, resulting in poor communication (Attree, 2001). Kim et al. (2008) further examined the challenges of discussing sexual history in Asian contexts, conducting research in Korea. About 25% of the interviewed patients reported discomfort in sharing sexual concerns with male doctors due to the doctors' gender, making communication highly ineffective.

Confucian Family-Centred Values: The Varying Level of Patient Involvement Across the Asian Region

The issue surrounding the level of involvement of patients' relatives is a recurring and vital theme in healthcare communication within East Asian contexts. Traditionally, in Chinese culture, families play a central role in making decisions about patients' treatments. Lin et al. (2016) highlighted this by studying 12 patients and their families involved in surgical decisions. They found that patients often refrained from expressing discomfort directly to doctors, leaving family members to give informed consent and participate in decision-making. This dynamic reflects a doctor-dominated communication pattern in China, consistent with Confucian values (Cong, 2004).

However, given Hong Kong's cultural diversity, researchers used an interdisciplinary approach to explore adapting Western patient-centred models (Pun et al., 2018). Unlike mainland Chinese patients, Wong et al. (2012) found that developing an advance directive for patients with advanced malignancy was feasible. By actively involving patients in their EOL arrangements, healthcare professionals align their goals with those of the patients and their families, facilitating patient participation in decision-making. Compared to findings in Japan, there appears to be an increasing trend towards greater patient involvement in decision-making. Japanese researchers noted that nurses were tasked with finding medical solutions that respected Japanese values of harmony and respect (Konishi et al., 2009; Konishi & Davis, 1999), thereby helping to mediate between patients and their families (Toda et al., 2015). This suggests that healthcare practices in Hong Kong and Japan are increasingly incorporating elements of Western patient-centred models, highlighting the need for further interdisciplinary research on the convergence between East Asian and Western healthcare communication approaches.

Elements That Impact the Quality of Medical Care in East Asia Cultural Sensitivity: Patients' and Families' Attitudes Towards EOL Discussions

East Asian settings call for more interdisciplinary research due to the distinct approaches taken by East Asian physicians in treating terminal patients compared to their Western counterparts. The review article by Pun et al. (2018) examined Cheng et al.'s (2015) cross-cultural survey of palliative care physicians in Japan, Korea, and Taiwan. It not only addressed East Asian contexts broadly but also highlighted cultural differences among East Asian countries that result in varying EOL practices. For example, the survey revealed that approximately 70% of Taiwanese clinicians face challenges with families' reluctance to discuss EOL issues; in Taiwan and Korea, the most senior family member typically takes on the role of decision-maker when delivering bad news, and entire families are often present during deaths; in Japan, there is a preference for family members to care for the dying patient and clean the deceased's body themselves. In China, Zheng et al. (2015) explored the experiences of 28 oncology nurses caring for terminal cancer patients, indicating that cultural sensitivity significantly impacts the quality of healthcare communication with both patients and their families. Although nurses were dedicated to providing high-quality EOL care, Zheng et al. (2015) noted the emotional toll such care took on them. The research team also compared these findings with another study, suggesting that Chinese nurses are not adequately trained in coping strategies when dealing with dying patients (Mak et al., 2013).

Asian Communication Preferences: Influences on Patients' Trust, Decision-Making Processes, and Level of Satisfaction

By conducting an interdisciplinary thematic analysis, the research team recognized the crucial role that trust plays in the effectiveness of doctor-patient interactions. Pun et al. (2018) highlighted Tang's research, which demonstrated that Chinese patients' trust in their doctors significantly impacts their overall satisfaction with the medical services and encounters they receive (Tang, 2011). The team then compared these findings to the situation in Hong Kong. As per Hui and Pun et al. (2015), the trust patients have in their doctors is closely linked to their satisfaction with clinical interactions and services. In South Korea, Lee et al. (2013) found that primary outcomes tend to improve when patients maintain longer-term relationships with their primary care practitioners (Lee et al., 2013).

Additionally, the number of hospital complaints tends to lower when there is increased engagement between clinicians and patients. Zhang et al. (2011), for example, observed that the attitudes of patients and their families towards doctors and hospitals were significant factors in deciding whether to file malpractice lawsuits in Taiwan. The research team's interdisciplinary study revealed differences in patient expectations regarding involvement in decision-making across various East Asian regions. For example, Chinese patients generally prefer a clinician-led, authoritative communication model, whereas those in Hong Kong often seek a more active role in their care (Pun et al., 2018). To further explore the contrast between preferences of Chinese and Hong Kong patients, the research team analysed Zhang et al.'s (2011) findings, which showed that Chinese patients typically adopt a passive approach to medical decision-making. Conversely, Hong Kong patients often play a more proactive role, emphasizing their needs while also recognizing their doctors' expertise (Henderson & Chien, 2007), potentially due to their focus on reassurance, patient confidentiality, and individualism (Arthur et al., 2004).

The research team investigated how South Korea's cultural context affects clinician-patient interactions from an interdisciplinary perspective. The core societal values in South Korea are deeply influenced by Confucianism (Kim et al., 2008), which creates parallels with clinician-patient dynamics in China. According to literature reviewed by Chang et al. (2013), South Korean doctors tend to display less empathy in patient communication (Kim et al., 2008). Chang et al.'s (2013) analysis of communication in rehabilitation settings revealed that fewer than 9% of patient utterances were categorized as active communication behaviours, with about half of the patients not asking any questions.

The team also examined Noh et al.'s (2009) study on information-seeking behaviours among Korean women with cervical cancer. It was found that only 41.7% of these patients sought information about their condition, primarily driven by their need for it. By comparing and analysing these three studies, the research team highlighted how traditional cultural values impact patient participation, including their reluctance to share medical history or seek additional information from doctors (Cong, 2004). The findings indicate that patient involvement in decision-making significantly influences their satisfaction, such as the frequency of communication with doctors and the availability of doctors to discuss critical health concerns after leaving the hospital (Pun et al., 2018).

Is Patient-Centred Care Truly Implemented in Real Life?

In Hong Kong, the Hospital Authority, which governs and oversees the management of local public hospitals, has emphasized patient-centred care as a fundamental value by promoting effective "two-way communication" as an essential strategy for clinicians to understand and address patient needs (Hong Kong Hospital Authority, 2013). Nevertheless, research indicates that this model may not fully suit the local context, as issues such as communication breakdowns between clinicians and patients or among clinicians have led to patient dissatisfaction (Griffiths & Yeoh, 2011; Hong Kong Hospital Authority, 2014). Doctors in Hong Kong often prioritize physical over emotional and social needs, leading patients to feel their overall care is neglected (Yam & Rossiter, 2000). Similarly, nurses were noted for focusing on tasks rather than interpersonal aspects of care (Pun et al., 2016).

To better understand Hong Kong patients' views on effective medical communication, the research team conducted interdisciplinary studies and observed medical settings. Pun et al. (2018) found that certain practices enhance patient-centred communication, such as small gestures, positive body language, and showing sincerity, which reflect sensitivity to patients' needs (Yam & Rossiter, 2000). Another study by Zayts and Kang (2009) emphasized the importance of interactive information delivery, comprehensive medical and psycho-social support, and empathetic behaviours from clinicians during diagnoses and treatments.

In addition to Hong Kong, the research team compared local findings with Japanese studies to evaluate trends in patient-centred approaches in East Asian medical settings. Ohtaki et al. (2003) noted that Japanese medical consultations were generally shorter, while physical exams and diagnostic discussions were more prolonged compared to those of the United States. Goto et al. (2015) analysed 16 consultations between family doctors and patients in Japan, finding that doctors who listened more to patients' stories engaged more actively in history-taking and diagnostics. Further supporting this trend, Takayama et al. (2001) found that patients who were satisfied with their doctors' communication styles were less anxious, even when receiving unfavourable results.

Multilingual and Multidisciplinary Communication in Asian Medical Care

To examine the medical context of Hong Kong more closely, which is a primary focus of this book, the research team's analysis of Hong Kong as a case study is crucial for understanding multilingual care environments. In Hong Kong, Chinese-speaking nurses are trained in Western theories, communicative models, and strategies. Although their education is conducted in English, these nurses interact with patients in Cantonese or Mandarin, their native languages, within the framework of traditional Chinese cultural practices (Pun et al., 2018). Consequently, these nurses often emphasize physical comfort, as their communication models are rooted in Western approaches (Yam et al., 2001).

The interdisciplinary review conducted by the research team demonstrated a cross-disciplinary perspective, examining trilingual environments and the quality of clinician-patient communication in emergency rooms. This included studying the communicative behaviours and knowledge of various stakeholders such as clinicians, nurses, educators, linguists, and communication researchers. Slade et al. found that communication in a local ER was complicated due to several contextual factors (Slade et al., 2015): (1) complex communication networks involving multiple clinicians interacting with each patient; (2) the necessity for cross-disciplinary, cross-level, cross-cultural, and multilingual collaboration in high-stress environments; (3) the requirement for clinicians to switch between Cantonese, Mandarin, and English; (4) high patient loads, limited time for procedures, and staff shortages.

Building on these identified principles, the research team reviewed Pun et al.'s (2016) study on clinicians' perceptions of communication challenges in a trilingual ED. Approximately half of the clinicians reported concerns about information being omitted or distorted during repeated translation. Additionally, 83% noted communication issues at triage, while over 40% experienced difficulties with documenting medical information. Long working hours were also reported to negatively affect communication, with 50% of clinicians noting reduced motivation to listen to patients during consultations.

This final subtheme highlighted by the research team's interdisciplinary review underscores how linguistic complexity in Hong Kong hospitals impacts the effectiveness of medical communication in local ERs. The team recommended further research into issues such as repeated translation of medical information, documentation challenges, and culturally specific professional pressures. Such studies could potentially address problems like misunderstandings and communication gaps between patients and clinicians and among clinicians themselves.

* * *

This chapter has examined prior research in applied linguistics and provided insights into the methodology of interdisciplinary research in healthcare contexts in Asia. By outlining the essential steps for conducting interdisciplinary studies and reviewing relevant literature, it highlights the importance and potential of extending research beyond traditional disciplinary boundaries to understand the intricacies of the Asian context, and, specifically, Hong Kong's trilingual environment.

Crossing disciplinary boundaries allows researchers to gain new insights by integrating various themes, such as those found in East Asian healthcare communication. While conflicts between different theoretical perspectives are inevitable, these disagreements should be viewed as valuable discoveries (Rhoten & Parker, 2004), as they help address unresolved and complex research issues (Campbell, 2005). By recognizing potential conflicts between different fields of knowledge and drawing from various disciplines, applied linguistics researchers can establish a shared framework for academic understanding, thereby advancing their exploration of intricate language-related issues and patterns in diverse contexts.

References

Arthur, D., Chong, C., Rujkorakarn, D., Wong, D., & Wongpanarak, N. (2004). A profile of the caring attributes of Hong Kong and Thailand psychiatric nurses. *International Journal of Mental Health Nursing, 13*(2), 100–106.

Attree, M. (2001). Patients' and relatives' experiences and perspectives of 'good' and 'not so good' quality care. *Journal of Advanced Nursing, 33*(4), 456–466.

Bracken, L. J., & Oughton, E. A. (2006). 'What do you mean?' The importance of language in developing interdisciplinary research. *Transactions of the Institute of British Geographers, 31*(3), 371–382.

Brookes, G., & Hunt, D. (2021). *Analysing Health Communication Discourse Approaches*. Palgrave Macmillan.

Campbell, L. M. (2005). Overcoming obstacles to interdisciplinary research. *Conservation Biology, 19*(2), 574–577.

Chang, C. L., Park, B. K., & Kim, S. S. (2013). Conversational analysis of medical discourse in rehabilitation: A study in Korea. *The Journal of Spinal Cord Medicine, 36*(1), 24–30.

Cheng, S. Y., Suh, S. Y., Morita, T., Oyama, Y., Chiu, T. Y., Koh, S. J., Kim, H. S., Hwang, S. J., Yoshie, T., & Tsuneto, S. (2015). A cross-cultural study on behaviors when death is approaching in east Asian countries: What are the physician-perceived common beliefs and practices? *Medicine (Baltimore), 94*(39), e1573.

Cicourel, A. V. (1999). The interaction of cognitive and cultural models in health care delivery. In I. S. Sarangi & C. Roberts (Eds.), *Talk Work and Institutional Order: Discourse in Medical, Mediation and Management Settings* (pp. 183–226). De Gruyter.

Cong, Y. (2004). Doctor-family-patient relationship: The Chinese paradigm of informed consent. *The Journal of Medicine and Philosophy, 29*(2), 149–178.

Dong, F., Zheng, R., Chen, X., Wang, Y., Zhou, H., & Sun, R. (2016). Caring for dying cancer patients in the Chinese cultural context: A qualitative study from the perspectives of physicians and nurses. *European Journal of Oncology Nursing, 21*, 189–196.

Goto, M., Yokoya, S., Takemura, Y., Gayle, A. A., & Tsuda, T. (2015). Describing the factors that influence the process of making a shared-agenda in Japanese family physician consultations: A qualitative study. *Asia Pacific Family Medicine, 14*(1), 6.

Griffiths, S., & Yeoh, E. (2011). Patient Satisfaction Survey 2010.

Henderson, A., & Chien, W. T. (2007). Health beliefs and expectations implicit in decision-making in a Hong Kong Chinese surgical population. *Journal of Clinical Nursing, 16*(3), 603–609.

Hong Kong Hospital Authority. (2013). *Vision, Missions & Values*. Retrieved from http://www.ha.org.hk

Hong Kong Hospital Authority. (2014). *Annual Report on Sentinel and Serious Untoward Events*. Retrieved from http://www.ha.org.hk/haho/ho/psrm/ECOPYSEREPORT2014.PDF

Hsiao, F. H., Klimidis, S., Minas, H., & Tan, E. S. (2006). Cultural attribution of mental health suffering in Chinese societies: The views of Chinese patients with mental illness and their caregivers. *Journal of Clinical Nursing, 15*(8), 998–1006.

Ishikawa, H., Hashimoto, H., Roter, D. L., Yamazaki, Y., Takayama, T., & Yano, E. (2005). Patient contribution to the medical dialogue and perceived patient-centeredness: An observational study in Japanese geriatric consultations. *Journal of General Internal Medicine, 20*(10), 906–910. https://doi.org/10.1111/j.1525-1497.2005.0200.x PMC

Jiang, L. L., Ruan, H., Xiang, X. J., & Jia, Q. (2015). Investigation and analysis of the caring attitude and behaviour of nurses in Shanghai, China. *International Journal of Nursing Practice, 21*(4), 426–432.

Kim, S. H., Lee, Y. M., & Park, J. T. (2008). Patients' perspectives on sexual history taking in Korea. *Patient Education and Counseling, 70*(3), 370–375.

Klein, J. T. (2008). Evaluation of interdisciplinary and transdisciplinary research: A literature review. *American Journal of Preventive Medicine, 35*(2), S116–S123.

Konishi, E., & Davis, A. J. (1999). Japanese nurses' perceptions about disclosure of information at the patients' end of life. *Nursing & Health Sciences, 1*(3), 179–187.

Konishi, E., Yahiro, M., Nakajima, N., & Ono, M. (2009). The Japanese value of harmony and nursing ethics. *Nursing Ethics, 16*(5), 625–636.

Lattuca, L. R. (2001). *Creating Interdisciplinarity: Interdisciplinary Research and Teaching among College and University Faculty*. Vanderbilt University Press.

Lee, J. H., Choi, Y. J., Lee, S. H., Sung, N. J., Kim, S. Y., & Hong, J. Y. (2013). Association of the length of doctor-patient relationship with primary care quality in seven family practices in Korea. *Journal of Korean Medical Science, 28*(4), 508–515.

Lin, M. L., Huang, C. T., & Chen, C. H. (2016). Reasons for family involvement in elective surgical decision-making in Taiwan: A qualitative study. *Journal of Clinical Nursing, 26*(13–14), 1967–1977.

Liu, J. E., Mok, E., & Wong, T. (2006). Caring in nursing: Investigating the meaning of caring from the perspective of cancer patients in Beijing, China. *Journal of Clinical Nursing, 15*(2), 188–196.

Mak, Y. W., Chiang, V. C., & Chui, W. T. (2013). Experiences and perceptions of nurses caring for dying patients and families in the acute medical admission setting. *International Journal of Palliative Nursing, 19*(9), 423–431.

Metzger, N., & Zare, R. N. (1999). Interdisciplinary research: From belief to reality. *Science, 283*, 642–643.

Noh, H. I., Lee, J. M., Yun, Y. H., Park, S. Y., Bae, D. S., Nam, N. J., et al. (2009). Cervical cancer patient information-seeking behaviours, information needs, and information sources in South Korea. *Supportive Care in Cancer, 17*(10), 1277–1283.

Ohtaki, S., Ohtaki, T., & Fetters, M. D. (2003). Doctor–patient communication: A comparison of the USA and Japan. *Family Practice, 20*(3), 276–282.

Porter, A. L., Roessner, J. D., Cohen, A. S., & Perreault, M. (2006). Interdisciplinary research: Meaning, metrics and nurture. *Research Evaluation, 15*(3), 187–195.

Pun, J., Matthiessen, C. M. I. M., Slade, D., & Murray, K. (2015). Factors affecting communication in emergency departments: Doctors and nurses' perceptions of communication in a trilingual ED in Hong Kong. *International Journal of Emergency Medicine, 8*, 48.

Pun, J., Chan, E. A., Matthiessen, C. M. I. M., Slade, D., & Murray, K. (2016). Clinicians' perceptions of communication challenges in a trilingual emergency department. *Journal of Clinical Nursing, 26*, 3396–3407.

Pun, J., Chan, E. A., Wang, S., & Slade, D. (2018). Health professional-patient communication practices in East Asia: An integrative review of an emerging field of research and practice in Hong Kong, South Korea, Japan, Taiwan, and Mainland China. *Patient Education and Counseling, 101*(7), 1193–1206.

Pun, J., Chan, E. A., Man, M., Eggins, S., & Slade, D. (2019). Pre- and post-evaluations of the effects of the connect, ask, respond and empathise (CARE) protocol on nursing handover: A case study of a bilingual hospital in Hong Kong. *Journal of Clinical Nursing, 28*, 3001.

Repko, A. F., Szostak, R., & Buchberger, M. P. (2016). *Introduction to Interdisciplinary Studies*. Sage Publications.

Rhoten, D. (2004). Interdisciplinary research: Trend or transition. *Items and Issues, 5*(1–2), 6–11.

Rhoten, D., & Parker, A. (2004). Risks and rewards of an interdisciplinary research path. *Science, 306*, 2046.

Roberts, C., & Sarangi, S. (1999). In S. Sarangi & C. Roberts (Eds.), *Talk, Work and Institutional Order: Discourse in Medical, Mediation and Management Settings*. De Gruyter.

Samovar, L., Porter, R. E., & Stefani, L. A. (1998). *Communication Between Cultures*. Wadsworth.
Siu, J. Y. M. (2015). Communicating under medical patriarchy: Gendered doctor-patient communication between female patients with overactive bladder and male urologists in Hong Kong. *BMC Women's Health, 15*(1), 44.
Slade, D., Chandler, E., Pun, J., et al. (2015). Effective healthcare worker-patient communication in Hong Kong accident & emergency departments. *Hong Kong Journal of Emergency Medicine, 22*(2), 69–83.
Stern, H. H., Stern, H. H., Tarone, E. E., Stern, H., & Yule, G. (1983). *Fundamental Concepts of Language Teaching: Historical and Interdisciplinary Perspectives on Applied Linguistic Research*. Oxford University Press.
Takayama, T., Yamazaki, Y., & Katsumata, N. (2001). Relationship between outpatients' perceptions of physicians' communication styles and patients' anxiety levels in a Japanese oncology setting. *Social Science & Medicine, 53*(10), 1335–1350.
Tang, L. (2011). The influences of patient's trust in medical service and attitude towards health policy on patient's overall satisfaction with medical service and sub satisfaction in China. *BMC Public Health, 11*(1), 1.
Toda, Y., Sakamoto, M., Tagaya, A., Takahashi, M., & Davis, A. J. (2015). Patient advocacy: Japanese psychiatric nurses recognizing necessity for intervention. *Nursing Ethics, 22*(7), 765–777.
Van Noorden, R. (2015). Interdisciplinary research by the numbers. *Nature News, 525*(7569), 306.
Varey, R. J. (1995). Internal marketing: A review and some interdisciplinary research challenges. *International Journal of Service Industry Management, 6*(1), 40–63.
Wang, Q. (2010). *Doctor-patient communication and patient satisfaction: A cross-cultural comparative study between China and the US.* (Unpublished doctoral dissertation). Purdue University.
Wong, S. Y., Lo, S. H., Chan, C. H., Chui, H. S., Sze, W. K., & Tung, Y. (2012). Is it feasible to discuss an advance directive with a Chinese patient with advanced malignancy? A prospective cohort study. *Hong Kong Medical Journal, 18*(3), 178–185.
Yam, B. M. C., & Rossiter, J. C. (2000). Caring in nursing: Perceptions of Hong Kong nurses. *Journal of Clinical Nursing, 9*(2), 293–302. https://doi.org/10.1046/j.1365-2702.2000.00349.x Wiley Online Library
Yam, B., Rossiter, J. C., & Cheung, K. (2001). Caring for dying infants: Experiences of neonatal intensive care nurses in Hong Kong. *Journal of Clinical Nursing, 10*(5), 651–659.

Yin, C. P., Hsu, C. W., Kuo, F. Y., & Huang, Y. T. (2012). A study of politeness strategies adopted in pediatric clinics in Taiwan. *Health Communication, 27*(6), 533–545.

Zayts, O., & Kang, M. A. (2009). "So, what test do you prefer?" Negotiating politic behaviour in an L2 prenatal genetic counselling setting in Hong Kong. *Journal of Politeness Research, 5*(1), 33–51. https://doi.org/10.1515/JPLR.2009.003

Zhang, Y., Su, H., Shang, L., Li, D., Wang, R., Zhang, R., & Xu, Y. (2011). Preferences and perceived involvement in treatment decision making among Chinese patients with chronic hepatitis. *Medical Decision Making, 31*(2), 245–253.

Zheng, R. S., Guo, Q. H., Dong, F. Q., & Owens, R. G. (2015). Chinese oncology nurses' experience on caring for dying patients who are on their final days: A qualitative study. *International Journal of Nursing Studies, 52*(1), 288–296.

Zhu, H. (2014). *Exploring Intercultural Communication: Language in Action*. Routledge.

3

Understanding Communication in Critical Care: Clinicians' and Patients' Perspectives

The Significance of Effective Communication in High-Risk Medical Settings

Effective medical communication is acknowledged as an important element globally for clinicians to make accurate diagnoses and develop appropriate treatment plans. On an interpersonal level, strong communication in healthcare settings helps patients understand critical medical information, fostering trust and enhancing their overall care experience (Health Canada, 2004). Various international studies have shown that poor or inaccurate clinical communication can compromise patient safety, particularly in high-risk environments like Intensive Care Units (ICUs) as well as Emergency Departments (EDs) (Lingard et al., 2004; Sutcliffe et al., 2004; Apker et al., 2007; Kachalia et al., 2007; Cheung et al., 2010; Slade et al., 2011a, 2011b). These studies highlighted that ineffective communication in these settings could lead to negative patient outcomes, including severe conditions or fatalities and compromised healthcare service quality like delayed care, misdiagnoses, and inappropriate treatments (Chisholm et al., 2000; Coiera et al., 2002; Ye et al., 2007; Cheung et al., 2010; Evans, 2015).

J. Pun, *Exploring and Teaching Healthcare Communication*,
https://doi.org/10.1007/978-3-031-08675-5_3

In light of these challenges, this chapter reviews three studies conducted in Hong Kong that involved interviews with ICU clinicians, mechanically ventilated (MV) patients, and ED clinicians, aiming to provide a broader perspective within a culturally and lingually diverse Asian context. The chapter begins by examining how ICU healthcare professionals perceive communication openness in a Hong Kong hospital and identifies the communication barriers they encounter. It explores their interactions within the ICU and across different departments, offering insights into the reasons for and methods to encourage a speak-up culture. Next, it addresses a research gap in understanding the interactive needs of MV patients who are conscious but unable to communicate verbally. This includes excerpts from interviews with ten former MV patients who had been in a multidisciplinary ICU for at least 24 hours, using the stimulated recall technique. It reveals the varied communication needs of these patients that extend beyond task-related topics (Leung et al., 2018), such as (1) medical discussions with healthcare providers, (2) communication with family members for support and guidance, (3) expressing their own requests and plans, (4) sharing feelings and perspectives on treatment, and (5) conveying psycho-emotional needs.

The chapter also discusses a study of an ED in Hong Kong to broaden the understanding of healthcare communication in high-risk Asian contexts. The final section narrows down its focus to the unique communication issues in Hong Kong's EDs, particularly the challenges of navigating trilingual interactions in a multicultural context. The findings are based on 28 interviews with local ED doctors and nurses, revealing linguistic challenges in shared decision-making and communication during trilingual clinical interactions.

What Benefits Does the Speak-Up Culture Bring to Patients in ICUs?

Ayoko (2007) defined "communication openness" as the comfort level individuals experience when verbally interacting with each other and the degree to which they achieve mutual understanding in conversation. This concept has since been linked with trust, active listening, honesty, and support. Rogers et al. (2007) expanded on Ayoko's definition by stating that communication openness involves behaviours related to the exchange of messages among superiors, subordinates, and peers. Within a medical context, Nolan (2000) suggested that fostering an environment where clinicians feel secure enough to speak freely is crucial for reducing patient safety risks. Ineffective communication and poor teamwork can jeopardize patient safety (Leonard et al., 2004). Studies by Lyndon et al. (2012) and Schwappach and Gehring (2014) described speaking up as a process where healthcare professionals voice their concerns about patient safety by posing immediate questions, sharing their views, or providing information until a clear resolution is reached, especially in cases where their superiors may have missed some information or made errors (Entwistle et al., 2010). Unfortunately, many healthcare professionals, particularly those in junior positions, tend to remain silent and hesitate to speak up even when patient safety is compromised due to medical mistakes (Morrison & Milliken, 2003).

Ensuring that clinicians are empowered to voice their concerns is key to preventing medical errors and eliminating risks to patient safety. Hospitals must promote a sense of psychological safety among their staff, which involves creating an environment where clinicians can express their ideas, ask questions, raise issues, or identify mistakes without fear of embarrassment, criticism, or guilt, so they feel comfortable sharing their thoughts and taking risks to speak up (Eppich, 2015; Edmondson, 2012, 1999). In high-risk healthcare environments, behaviours that disrupt communication such as shouting or displaying condescension towards colleagues or juniors can threaten a clinician's sense of safety (Eppich, 2015). Some healthcare professionals hesitate to speak up because they worry their concerns may be seen as a lack of knowledge, negativity, incompetence, or even disruptive behaviour by their peers (Eppich, 2015; Edmondson, 2012).

To assess how safe clinicians feel about speaking up for their patients, researchers often examine their levels of communication openness. Factors influencing their willingness to speak up can be both individual and contextual. Many healthcare professionals find that hierarchical structures and interdisciplinary practices within hospitals discourage them from doing so (Schwappach & Gehring, 2014). A study by Carter et al. (2013) found that British clinicians considered it inappropriate to challenge their seniors, fearing negative repercussions such as damaged relationships. The decision to speak up is influenced by various factors, including individual characteristics like tenure, work factors such as job structure, organizational culture, available data, and external pressures. Luong et al. (2009) also found that nurses and managers from traditional Asian family backgrounds tend to be less inclined to speak out. In Hong Kong, Law and Chan (2015) discovered a lack of understanding and trust between different generations of nurses, with senior clinicians rarely listening to nursing students' motivations to advocate for patient safety. Consequently, cultural factors often act as barriers to speaking up, particularly in Chinese clinical contexts.

ICU Clinicians' Perspectives in Hong Kong: Is It a Safe Environment for Speaking Up?

In a study about the culture of speaking up in a local ICU in Hong Kong, Ng et al. (2017) found that while the participants generally shared similar views on their levels of communication openness with colleagues, doctors often displayed a more favourable attitude towards communication openness than nurses in several respects. On the other hand, the nurses showed slightly more positive views towards nursing and medical leadership as well as the understanding of patient care objectives. The study also revealed differing perspectives among ICU doctors and nurses regarding the unit's speak-up culture. The main reasons for clinicians to speak up were typically to seek information or clarification. Other factors, such as hierarchical rank, language, and communication training, also influenced their willingness to speak up and related behaviours. Ng et al. (2017) examined ICU clinicians' views on their satisfaction with communication and teamwork within the unit, focusing on their perceptions of communication openness. Key aspects highlighted in the study included: (1) interactions between clinicians of different ranks and departments, (2) the timeliness of communication, (3) clinicians' comprehension of patient-care objectives, (4) the effectiveness of leadership within the team, and (5) the overall performance of the unit:

1. The participants generally viewed workplace communication positively, with the highest satisfaction levels observed in interactions between senior doctors and their colleagues across different ranks and departments. However, the nurses reported lower satisfaction regarding their communication with other team members.
2. The participating ICU clinicians expressed high satisfaction with the timeliness of communication, especially when it involved sharing patient care information, but nurses were less satisfied than doctors in this regard.
3. Overall, clinicians had a somewhat positive view of their understanding of patient care goals, including care plans, their own roles in implementing these plans, and potential risks to patient safety.
4. Compared to other aspects, participants were slightly less satisfied with the leadership within the ICU.
5. The clinicians also felt that the overall effectiveness of the unit was ideal.

Ng et al. (2017) observed slight positive correlations between ICU staff who had undergone communication training and their capacity for open dialogue and comprehension of patient-care objectives. Thus, providing adequate communication training to ICU clinicians is crucial, as it can enhance their reported ability to speak openly and grasp patient-care goals. The following sections include original views from local clinicians, which suggest ways to motivate their colleagues to speak up and strategies to do so.

Interviews: ICU Clinicians' Thoughts on the Promotion of Speak-Up Culture

What Are the Initiatives?

In the study by Ng et al. (2017), the senior ICU nurses reported that they would voice concerns regarding patient transfers, nursing handovers, and follow-up on treatments and medications. By doing so, they aimed to ensure effective information transfer for the benefit of their patients. One nurse mentioned employing a strategy of repeating the information received until they were confident that both they and their colleagues fully understood it.

> *[Nurses] might request additional information or ask for information to be clarified when information was lacking or unclear in the handover documents.*
>
> *[We would speak up] when we felt that we needed to know more about a case for effective follow-up or to clarify the current stage reached in the prescribed clinical treatment for the patient.*

The participating doctors tended to speak up primarily when they needed to gather more information or clarify messages, particularly during handovers, shift changes, or decision-making processes related to patient care. This practice helped ensure that treatments continued smoothly and that they had all the necessary information for making decisions about patient management. As a result, both ICU doctors and nurses would most commonly speak up to seek or clarify information. Very few would raise concerns for 'classical' reasons, such as identifying errors (like possible misdiagnoses or unsuitable treatments) or pointing out rule violations or deviations from standard procedures.

Things That Encourage ICU Clinicians to Speak Up

In the study by Ng et al. (2017), all interviewed ICU doctors and nurses believed that the unit effectively encouraged them to speak up when necessary, which may be linked to their tendency to engage in speak-up practices. They expressed similar opinions about the factors that would promote a speak-up culture within the unit: Their familiarity with the ICU patients' information and conditions in the ICU affects their willingness to speak up:

1. Their willingness to speak up was influenced by how well they knew the patients' information and conditions in the ICU.
2. They felt more comfortable speaking up if there were no strict hierarchies and if they had opportunities to share their perspectives, regardless of their rank or speciality.
3. They wanted more chances to ask questions and participate in medical discussions, which could be facilitated by minimizing conflicts between colleagues of different ranks. Trust could be fostered if everyone in the team showed respect, especially towards those familiar with a patient's case and willing to discuss any related issues.

Hierarchies and interpersonal conflicts were identified as significant factors that created tension and hindered communication within the team, leading to uncertainty about speaking up for patient safety. Some nurses mentioned that the main motivation for speaking up in critical situations was the desire to be seen as having equal professional status, without being constrained by the hierarchical structure:

> *We should listen to staff who spend the most time by the bedside of the patients, as nurses will clearly know the clinical development of the patients.*

Allocating Resources for Speak-Up Training

As previously mentioned, training sessions can effectively promote a culture of speaking up in the ICU. However, many participants in Ng et al.'s (2017) study were unaware of the communication training sessions provided by the Hospital Authority, which were designed to encourage them to speak up. Clinicians who had undergone crew resource management (CRM) training mentioned that the current programmes mainly emphasized team dynamics and strong leadership in high-pressure situations. They observed, however, a shortage of courses that support communication between clinicians during their routine daily tasks.

How to Speak Up Across Ranks Within the Unit and with Other Disciplines

As observed, hierarchical structures frequently obstruct clinicians' ability to speak up globally. Ng et al. (2017) found that this issue was also prevalent among ICU clinicians in Hong Kong. During interviews, nursing staff revealed they would only speak up to doctors when it was crucial for addressing patient cases, treatments, and medications. Nurses were generally more inclined to voice concerns than doctors. However, it was difficult for them to speak up to doctors, who often issued instructions that nurses simply followed. ICU doctors tended to engage with nurses only in very urgent situations. Additionally, doctors were usually occupied with their responsibilities, leaving nurses with limited opportunities for interaction. Consequently, ICU nurses commonly sought advice from the head nurse or asked the nurse-in-charge to relay their questions to the appropriate doctor.

Interdisciplinary communication emerged as another crucial element impacting both patient safety and the overall efficiency of the unit. Clinicians involved in the study considered it vital to engage with external disciplines such as ED colleagues and various medical and surgical teams during patient care. For instance, ICU doctors needed to verify specific medical details with colleagues from other departments, such as checking patient medications. However, the participants observed that the culture of speaking up across disciplines was rather lacking. Many junior doctors struggled to communicate with colleagues from other departments regarding patient management, feeling they had limited influence in decision-making. They also identified a hierarchical structure in these interdisciplinary interactions; for example, they were often instructed to communicate only with peers of similar rank or experience levels by phone. It was generally considered improper for junior staff to contact senior colleagues from other disciplines directly.

To address communication challenges, the participating ICU doctors and nurses emphasized the need for all clinicians to show greater patience and respect towards each other, including junior colleagues who might have specialized expertise, particularly when managing patients outside their own areas of specialization. The participants highlighted the value of actively listening to and striving to understand the perspectives of their colleagues. They also believed it was beneficial to encourage experienced professionals to voice their insights and serve as mentors to junior staff.

Additionally, the participants provided suggestions on improving speak-up practices at various levels within the unit and across different disciplines. They shared strategies on how junior clinicians could effectively communicate with their senior colleagues:

> *Junior doctors will speak up only when they have a strong, justified opinion or to clarify information related to patient harm. Senior doctors will speak up during a handover when they have more perceived role space through an understanding of their role contribution in providing a different opinion within a joint-team collaborative decision.*

Some interviewees believed that senior doctors had more opportunity to voice their opinions during patient-care decision-making due to their higher authority. Nonetheless, a senior doctor interviewed also recognized the importance of fostering a culture of speaking up within the unit, as even senior staff can make errors.

Some senior nurses noted that their junior counterparts were often quite reserved when asking questions during handovers. They expressed a willingness to create opportunities for junior staff to seek clarification or receive guidance on unfamiliar situations. Typically, junior nurses with less than a year of experience need time to become accustomed to medical terminology specific to the unit, learn handover procedures, and understand potential patient safety risks (Ng et al., 2017). Thus, the senior nurses emphasized the importance of junior nurses asking questions during handovers when they encountered unclear information.

Language and Cultural Norms: Accommodating Chinese Values

In Ng et al.'s (2017) study, ICU nurses and doctors employed various language strategies when speaking up. The nurses noted that many ICU staff members overlooked the importance of language use, focusing instead on medical concerns. They agreed that speaking up practices varied according to individual communication styles, resulting in a lack of awareness about specific expressions for this purpose. A senior nurse highlighted the need to use a non-threatening tone to make colleagues more comfortable in critical situations.

Some doctors mentioned that they would base their speak-up moments on factual descriptions derived from their observations. They emphasized the importance of providing adequate background information before presenting their points and allowing others to evaluate these points. This approach corresponds with the ISBAR framework (Introduction, Situation, Background, Assessment, and Recommendation) used in medical handovers, which is endorsed in both local and international hospitals (Thompson et al., 2011). Additionally, the doctors found open-ended questions helpful for making inquiries, as this method encourages a broader discussion among the ICU team rather than making immediate judgments. Non-verbal cues, such as eye contact, were also suggested to signal the need for questions and to prompt junior colleagues to participate.

Junior ICU doctors reported that indirect communication strategies were particularly effective. Instead of addressing senior clinicians directly, they would involve the entire team in reviewing lab reports and clinical images like X-rays, thereby drawing attention to potentially overlooked medical information. These indirect communication strategies reflect the Chinese cultural emphasis on maintaining harmony, which allows clinicians to navigate role boundaries flexibly without undermining others' status or face (Edmondson, 1999).

A Summarized Guide to Speaking Up in High-Risk Chinese Medical Settings

To foster a speak-up culture in a Chinese medical context, the interviewed ICU clinicians in Ng et al.'s (2017) study provided the following recommendations:

1. Speak sincerely when addressing clinicians of varying ranks or experience levels.
2. Ensure and reach a shared understanding of the latest patient information among all members involved in decision-making, and communicate clearly so that everyone can easily grasp and discuss the details.
3. Establish a common language for speaking up within the unit.
4. Encourage speak-up practices between junior and senior clinicians.
5. Develop a non-blaming environment to make junior doctors feel safe when speaking up. Discourage retaliatory practices, as they can deter juniors from reporting minor issues.
6. Avoid using specific ICU jargon with unique meanings that are only understood within a single hospital.

Patients' Perspectives: How to Facilitate Clinicians' Understanding of the Needs of Their MV Patients?

In addition to clinicians, patients undergoing MV in high-risk environments often face communication challenges. Although tracheal intubation and MV are crucial for many ICU patients, those on MV struggle to verbally communicate. These patients, typically in critical conditions, experience significant frustration when they are unable to express themselves. Given current practices of light sedation or daily sedation interruptions, ICU patients may spend extended periods conscious but unable to speak (Kress et al., 2000; Mehta et al., 2012). Khalaila et al. (2011) reported that 40–80% of patients receiving invasive ventilation found communication to be moderately to extremely difficult, with 60% feeling highly frustrated by unmet communication needs (Patak et al., 2004; Happ et al., 2011).

Recent research indicated that traditional communication between patients and clinicians, as well as between patients and their families, is considered essential but often inadequate in quality for all involved (Leathart, 1994; Institute of Medicine Committee, 2001; Constand et al., 2014; Magnus & Turkington, 2006; Happ et al., 2004; Myhren et al., 2009; Ashworth, 1980; Menzel, 1998; Broyles et al., 2012; Carroll, 2004; Tembo et al., 2015). ICU clinicians typically prioritize discussions about physical symptoms and care tasks (Happ et al., 2004; Ashworth, 1980). Consequently, the needs of MV patients can be overlooked, leading to misunderstandings. Patients may be forced to simplify their communication due to these barriers (Carroll, 2004). The inability to communicate effectively can cause distress, anxiety, anger, fear, a sense of losing control, feeling imprisoned, depersonalized, and socially isolated, potentially resulting in long-term effects such as post-intensive care anxiety or even depression (Khalaila et al., 2011; Patak et al., 2004; Happ et al., 2011; Myhren et al., 2009; Tembo et al., 2015; Carroll, 2007; Bergbom-Engberg, 1989).

MV Patients' Range of Communication Needs

Leung et al. (2018) used the stimulated recall method and conducted interviews with MV patients to examine their communication needs. They found that these needs were multifaceted, covering areas such as medical conversations with ICU clinicians, expressing suffering and emotions, seeking support, making plans, and sharing personal viewpoints with family members. Many of these communication needs were not fully met. Consequently, it is crucial to develop ICU strategies that enable MV patients to engage in conversations about medical, non-medical, and psycho-emotional matters, rather than limiting communication to basic symptoms or task-related issues.

The patients expressed a desire to actively participate in discussions with their clinicians, including medical conversations. While some messages about physical discomfort were straightforward and easily understood by clinicians, others were more intricate. For instance, patients sometimes wanted to share their personal opinions on treatment decisions or express their wish to limit therapy. Leung et al. (2018) highlighted that ICU clinicians need to be highly attuned to their MV patients' emotional states and address these concerns appropriately, whether they involve personal opinions or temporary emotional responses.

Additionally, the interviewed MV patients indicated a wish to discuss their conditions with family members and maintain connections with both family and friends. They wanted the opportunity to exchange thoughts, feel supported, and show emotions such as love, gratitude, and regret.

Suggested Tools and Strategies to Actively Involve MV Patients in Communication

Leung et al. (2018) explored various communication tools and strategies used by ICU clinicians with MV patients in Hong Kong. They classified these methods into two main categories: (1) natural techniques such as mouthing words, nodding, facial expressions as well as body language, and (2) augmented alternative communication tools like writing, typing, communication boards, alphabet boards, and advanced electronic devices. While natural methods are straightforward, they are limited in conveying complex messages, often leaving MV patients and their caregivers frustrated and struggling to communicate effectively (Broyles et al., 2012).

To address this, communication boards with pre-set lists of content enable MV patients to indicate their needs by touching or pointing. In Hong Kong, options include boards from the Hong Kong Society of Critical Care and the Vidatak EZ Board, as well as digital apps like the "ICU Patient Communicator" (Hong Kong Society of Critical Care Medicine's ICU Communication Board in Traditional Chinese, 2010; Society of Critical Care Medicine, 2001; ten Hoorn et al., 2016; Patak et al., 2006). Leung et al. (2018) identified several types of content included in these tools: firstly, descriptions of physical sensations or brief emotional expressions like "sad," often supported by body diagrams and pain scales. Secondly, boards feature the phrase "I want" with options for physical tasks or environmental changes, such as turning off lights. Thirdly, options for requesting to see specific individuals, including doctors, nurses, or family members. Fourthly, pre-determined questions like "How am I doing?" and "What has happened?" Lastly, there are sections with alphabets and numbers for creating free-text messages. Although these tools facilitate basic communication, they fall short in addressing more complex interactions required for medical discussions, emotional support, and comprehensive conversations between ICU clinicians, MV patients, and their families (Broyles et al., 2012). The current methods of typing, writing, and using alphabet boards are often inadequate due to MV patients' physical limitations, including weakness, inability to perform tasks, oedema, and restricted mobility or vision.

MV patients frequently face psycho-emotional challenges during their periods of non-vocal communication. Leung et al. (2018) reported that patients often felt lonely and distressed when faced with potential death. Similar findings have been observed in other studies (Khalaila et al., 2011; Patak et al., 2004; Happ et al., 2011; Tembo et al., 2015). To develop effective communication tools for addressing these emotional struggles, the first step is to recognize and validate the patients' feelings.

Local Clinicians' Daily Challenges in High-Risk Medical Environments in Hong Kong

Lost in Translation

Similar to EDs in other parts of Asia and Europe, those in Hong Kong are predominantly trilingual. Cantonese, Mandarin, and English are commonly used, both in spoken and written forms. In these settings, clinicians often switch between these three languages due to their native language typically being Chinese, resulting in bilingual or even trilingual communication during daily tasks. This linguistic practice aligns with the official local languages and the use of English for higher education purposes (Chandler et al., 2015). In everyday operations, ED clinicians usually read and record medical details in English while speaking with patients in their native languages. During interactions among clinicians, they primarily use Cantonese with English medical terminology (Slade et al., 2015a, 2015b). This hybrid language usage, distinct from Standard English, can sometimes cause inconsistencies in medical records, requiring multiple translation steps throughout a patient's care journey (Matthiessen, 2013). Moreover, frequent code-switching by clinicians complicates patient comprehension, as patients may not understand all the languages being used (Slade et al., 2016). The intricate trilingual environment and the pressure of time constraints make accurate medical documentation difficult, often resulting in errors (Pun et al., 2015). Overall, communication in local EDs is frequently at risk.

Pun et al. (2015) conducted interviews with ED clinicians in Hong Kong and found that miscommunication was most likely to occur during patient handovers. The interviewed clinicians noted that errors were common, such as doctors providing incorrect verbal instructions and nurses confusing medications with similar-sounding English names. A senior ED doctor highlighted the potential risks to patient safety due to these communication issues:

> *Sometimes the [doctors] may give a verbal order . . . and maybe what the doctors ordered was not well-perceived by our staff. . . . And so it may lead to some misunderstanding in delivering – I mean a wrong dosage or wrong rate of infusions for the patient. And so this is one of the communication problems that I've observed . . . in the past 12 months.* (INT_Doc_1)

Another senior ED doctor mentioned that creating English medical notes often involved selectively summarizing what patients expressed in Cantonese:

> *Of course we have to condense a very long story into [something] concise. Because we just can't copy what the patients say. Even if they speak in English, we can't copy what they say.* (INT_Doc_5)

Regarding the explanation of medical information to patients, one doctor noted that communication problems frequently occurred when attempting to translate directly from written English to spoken Cantonese:

> *For some specific disease that we know in English, sometimes for some rare diseases it may be difficult for us to find the right Chinese term to explain to the patient.* (INT_Doc_2)

A senior doctor interviewed acknowledged that translation could result in omissions or alterations of medical details and explained the steps they and their colleagues took to address this issue:

> *Because we have [been] doing this for so many years, we try to closely relate those Cantonese things into the notes. But sometimes actually the Cantonese cannot be directly translated into the English. I think many colleagues will put the Chinese character inside the notes.* (INT_Doc_1)

These excerpts from the interviews highlight the trilingual environment and code-switching practices in local EDs, demonstrating how often communication barriers arise from such practices.

The Faulted Process of Medical Documentation

Almost half of the participants in Pun et al.'s (2015) research reported facing difficulties with communication while creating written medical records. They noted that each colleague had individual preferences for how to convey information, whether through written notes, verbal communication, or a combination of both. As a result, they found it challenging to anticipate how their colleagues would choose to communicate or when they might switch between methods. Due to this inconsistency, the interviewees had to rely on their own judgment to interpret the spoken or documented details about a patient's medical history and symptoms during handovers. One participant compared the communication process in the ED to "chaotic traffic," especially during handovers, where vital information could easily be omitted or altered.

Triage as a Point of Miscommunication: Problems with Time Limitations and the Lack of Manpower

Many of the ED clinicians interviewed in Pun et al.'s (2015) study stated that the most difficult moments for communication with colleagues and patients occurred during critical transition points in a patient's care. A senior doctor provided an example regarding the triage station:

> *I think the triage is the most high-pressure area in our department because the volume of [patients] is so . . . high. Sometimes there may be 30, 40, 60 patients waiting outside in the waiting hall to be seen by the doctor, so triage became a very convenient point for them to go to the triage nurse and ask 'What's happening here? And why am I waiting here so long?' And so I think problems can arise easily in the triage area, and communication is a very important tool to overcome those problems.* (INT_Doc_2)

Being different from other EDs, those in Hong Kong explicitly inform admitted patients of their triage categories. However, despite being aware of their categories, patients often endure long waiting times without adequate explanations from clinicians, which causes frustration. Serious problems can occur if a patient is placed in the wrong triage category. One senior doctor pointed out that severe consequences, such as worsening conditions or even death, can happen when a patient's condition is under-categorized:

> *We had a patient who was referred from a GP because of leg swelling. Actually, the GP had written in the referral notes that a clot inside the blood vessel was suspected. But it was inappropriately triaged and the patient was left waiting for two hours; and then the patient collapsed and finally died of lung–primary embolism.* (INT_Doc_3)

Effective communication could have prevented this tragic incident, but the clinicians responsible could be unaware of the problem at the triage stage. The interviewed doctor further explained that this patient's misclassification resulted from poor communication:

> *In terms of communication, maybe you are worried that [the triage staff] did not read the GP's letter carefully. We're not sure whether it was due to the time limitations or whether it was due to a lack of knowledge of this disease...* (INT_Doc_6)

These critical errors can cause distress for both patients' families and clinicians and can have serious implications for the hospitals involved. Without corrective measures, the factors that compromise communication in Hong Kong EDs may become embedded in routine medical practices (Pun et al., 2015).

Many ED clinicians in Hong Kong also deal with significant time constraints and heavy patient loads (Pun et al., 2015). According to Pun et al. (2015), the emergency department they examined typically involved two or more doctors briefly discussing patients during clinical handovers. The clinicians reported that, in these conversations, they often used short, informal sentences, spoken in Cantonese or a mix of Cantonese and English. During these handovers, they also took notes in English, using a condensed format with checkboxes that often overlooked details about changes in a patient's condition. One doctor noted that extensive documentation and thorough handovers were impractical in local EDs due to the high demand for emergency services and the resulting time constraints:

> *We have 600 patients a day.... So it would be very difficult for us to do a formal handover between doctors and nurses. So we just do some mini-handovers between the doctors themselves, and the nurses will also do some handovers among themselves.* (INT_Doc_7)

Limited Interpersonal Communication

As per Pun et al.'s (2015) study, although most of the participants acknowledged the importance of delivering patient-centred care and adhering to its principles, the high-pressure atmosphere of their workplace often left them feeling too overwhelmed or uneasy to engage actively in meaningful communication. Only a small portion of the interviewees felt able to demonstrate empathy towards their patients or take the time to reassure them about the quality of their care. Consequently, these ED clinicians limited patient involvement during consultations and decision-making about treatments, reducing the focus on showing empathy through interpersonal interactions (Slade et al., 2015a, 2015b). As a result, interpersonal communication skills and the support or training provided by local hospitals in this area need enhancement.

Recommendations on Tackling These Barriers and Fostering Trust Between Clinicians and Patients in High-Stress Environments

While there are various studies examining the nature and frequency of communication issues with patients who speak foreign languages (Frank, 2000; Bischoff et al., 2003; Hudelson & Vilpert, 2009) or come from culturally diverse backgrounds (Vasquez & Javier, 1991; Brooks, 1992; Timmins, 2002; Alegrıa et al., 2009), few have focused on how clinicians respond to communication needs in fast-paced, high-pressure and multilingual environments like EDs (Chandler et al., 2015; Pun et al., 2015; Slade et al., 2016). To address this gap, Slade et al. (2015a, 2015b) recommended communication training programmes tailored for ED healthcare providers, aiming to enhance the quality of medical communication, reduce patient complaints, prevent adverse events, and increase clinicians' confidence and job satisfaction. Slade et al. (2015a, 2015b) developed a communication framework to help ED clinicians in Hong Kong build rapport and explain medical concepts to patients. Building on this, Pun et al. (2015) investigated the discourse strategies employed by local ED clinicians to convey empathy. Their study expanded on Slade et al.'s (2015a, 2015b) findings to identify strategies for promoting effective medical knowledge sharing and decision-making, which include (1) creating opportunities for patients to share their stories; (2) recognizing patients' understanding and viewpoints regarding their health conditions; (3) using both medical and everyday language to clarify medical concepts; (4) communicating diagnoses and treatments in straightforward, direct language with patients. Table 3.1 provides further details on these strategies.

Table 3.1 Selected strategies for developing shared medical knowledge and decision-making

Communication strategies	Description	Talk
Creating the space for patients to talk about their stories	Opening the interaction for patient participation and allowing the space to tell their story	Dr: ==But do you feel unwell? P: Well ah … yesterday I felt … didn't feel quite well Dr: How so? Does it hurt?
Seeking and acknowledging patients' knowledge of and perspectives towards their medical conditions	Facilitate the knowledge-building process by eliciting and valuing patients' knowledge about their case and prior treatments	Dr: But do you feel sore today? You said you started to feel uncomfortable yesterday, how about today? Today
	Normalise patients' medical symptoms and concerns about what is happening to them	P: Here, I was leaning like this. Perhaps the pacemaker is here Dr: This isn't a concern, the metal is quite strong. If nothing's loose, then there's no problem P: No, right? I don't know. I got nervous, I, you know how nervous I am Dr: Well we did an electrocardiogram, tested things out, those-those signals are very normal
Talking to patients about their diagnoses and treatments using direct and clear terms	Limit technical language and explain terms that patients might not understand	Dr: Signals from the pacemaker are quite good P: Right Dr: Meaning that it hasn't lost its functions, things like that

(*continued*)

Table 3.1 (continued)

Communication strategies	Description	Talk
Talking to patients about their diagnoses and treatments using direct and clear terms	Provide patients with comprehensive explanations about diagnosis and clear instructions for on-going treatment or management plans	Dr: Now, let me prescribe you some meds P: Good, good, good Dr: Some ointment for you to apply on that bruised part, of your arm, huh? P: Mm. Meaning rub it on and it'll get better? Dr: Wait for it to fade, huh P: Wait for it to fade

Source: Slade et al., *Communicating in Hospital Emergency Departments* (London: Springer, 2015b)

Considering the traditional Chinese values that influence clinical environments in Hong Kong, ICU and ED clinicians are encouraged to prioritize human factors and core values, rather than solely focusing on conflict management. For ICU clinicians, speaking up is particularly essential to ensuring effective teamwork within their units. Additionally, they must recognize the wide range of both medical and non-medical communication needs of patients, especially those of MV patients.

This chapter also highlights the significant communication difficulties faced by clinicians in another high-risk environment: the EDs in Hong Kong. It discusses the various forms and challenges of communication in local EDs, such as frequent translation, inconsistent and inadequate medical documentation, and the pressures arising from a high-stress environment (e.g., extended working hours, heavy patient loads, and hierarchical tensions between junior and senior clinicians). A framework has been presented to help multilingual ED clinicians improve their communication skills by implementing patient-centred practices in Hong Kong.

References

Alegrıa, M., Sribney, W., Perez, D., Laderman, M., & Keefe, K. (2009). The role of patient activation on patient–provider communication and quality of care for US and foreign-born Latino patients. *Journal of General Internal Medicine, 24*, 534–541.

Apker, J., Mallak, L. A., & Gibson, S. C. (2007). Communicating in the "gray zone": Perceptions about emergency physician–hospitalist handoffs and patient safety. *Academic Emergency Medicine, 14*, 884–894.

Ashworth, P. (Ed.). (1980). *Care to Communicate: An Investigation Into Problems of Communication Between Patients and Nurses in Intensive Therapy Units* (Royal College of Nursing of UK Research Series). Whitefriars Press.

Ayoko, O. B. (2007). Communication openness, conflict events and reactions to conflict in culturally diverse workgroups. *Cross Cultural Management: An International Journal, 14*, 105–124.

Bergbom-Engberg, I. H. H. (1989). Assessment of patients' experience of discomforts during respiratory therapy. *Critical Care Medicine, 17*(10), 1068–1072.

Bischoff, A., Perneger, T. V., Bovier, P. A., Lou-tan, L., & Stalder, H. (2003). Improving communication between physicians and patients who speak a foreign language. *British Journal of General Practice, 53*, 541–546.

Brooks, T. R. (1992). Pitfalls in communication with Hispanic and African-American patients: Do translators help or harm? *Journal of the National Medical Association, 84*, 941.

Broyles, L. M., Tate, J. A., & Happ, M. B. (2012). Use of augmentative and alternative communication strategies by family members in the intensive care unit. *American Journal of Critical Care, 21*(2), e21–e22.

Carroll, S. M. (2004). Nonvocal ventilated patients perceptions of being understood. *Western Journal of Nursing Research, 26*(1), 85–103.

Carroll, S. M. (2007). Silent, slow lifeworld: The communication experience of nonvocal ventilated patients. *Qualitative Health Research, 17*(9), 1165–1677.

Carter, M., Thompson, N., Crampton, P., Morrow, G., Burford, B., Gray, C., & Illing, J. (2013). Workplace bullying in the UK NHS: A questionnaire and interview study on prevalence, impact and barriers to reporting. *BMJ Open, 3*, e002628.

Chandler, E., Slade, D., Pun, J., Lock, G., Matthiessen, C. M. I. M., Espindola, E., & Ng, C. (2015). Communication in Hong Kong accident & emergency departments: The clinicians' perspectives. *Global Qualitative Nursing Journal, 2*, 1–11.

Cheung, D. S., Kelly, J. J., Beach, C., et al. (2010). Improving handoffs in the emergency department. *Annals of Emergency Medicine, 55*(2), 171–180.

Chisholm, C. D., Collison, E. K., Nelson, D. R., & Cordell, W. H. (2000). Emergency department workplace interruptions: Are emergency physicians "interrupt-driven" and "multitasking"? *Academic Emergency Medicine, 7*, 1239–1243.

Coiera, E., Jayasuriya, R., Hardy, J., & Thrope, M. E. (2002). Communication loads on clinical staff in the emergency department. *Medical Journal of Australia, 176*, 415–418.

Constand, M. K., MacDermid, J. C., Dal Bello-Haas, V., & Law, M. (2014). Scoping review of patient-centered care approaches in healthcare. *BMC Health Services Research, 14*(271). https://doi.org/10.1186/1472-6963-14-271 macsphere.mcmaster.ca+6SCIRP+6SpringerLink+6

Edmondson, A. (1999). Psychological safety and learning behavior in work teams. *Administrative Science Quarterly, 44*(2), 350–383. https://doi.org/10.2307/2666999 content.lesaffaires.com+1Massachusetts Institute of Technology+1

Edmondson, A. C. (2012). *Teaming: How Organizations Learn, Innovate, and Compete in the Knowledge Economy*. A Wiley Imprint.

Entwistle, V. A., McCaughan, D., Watt, I. S., Birks, Y., Hall, J., Peat, M., Williams, B., & Wright, J. (2010). Speaking up about safety concerns: Multi-setting qualitative study of patients' views and experiences. *Quality & Safety in Health Care, 19*, e33.

Eppich, W. (2015). "Speaking up" for patient safety in the paediatric emergency department. *Clinical Paediatric Emergency Medicine, 16*(2), 83–89.

Evans, K. (2015). Emergency departments: Better safe than sorry? *Emergency Nurse, 23*, 20–22.

Frank, R. A. (2000). Medical communication: Non-native English-speaking patients and native English-speaking professionals. *English for Specific Purposes, 19*, 31–62.

Happ, M. B., Tuite, P., Dobbin, K., DiVirgilio-Thomas, D., & Kitutu, J. (2004). Communication ability, method, and content among nonspeaking non-surviving patients treated with mechanical ventilation in the intensive care unit. *American Journal of Critical Care, 13*(3), 210–220.

Happ, M. B., Garrett, K., Thomas, D. D., Tate, J., George, E., Houze, M., Radtke, J., & Sereika, S. (2011). Nurse-patient communication interactions in the intensive care unit. *American Journal of Critical Care, 20*(2), e28–e40.

Health Canada. (2004). *Interdisciplinary Education for Collaborative Patient-Centeredness: Research and Findings Report*. Health Canada.

Hong Kong Society of Critical Care Medicine's ICU Communication Board in Traditional Chinese. (2010). Retrieved from http://www.hksccm.org/index.php?option=com_content&view=article&id=2087:2010-oct-4-icu-communication-board&catid=241:communiation-tools&Itemid=9998&lang=en

Hudelson, P., & Vilpert, S. (2009). Overcoming language barriers with foreign-language speaking patients: A survey to investigate intra-hospital variation in attitudes and practices. *BioMed Central Health Services Research, 9*, 187.

Institute of Medicine Committee on Quality of Health Care in America (Ed.). (2001). *Crossing the Quality Chasm: A New Health System for the 21st Century*. National Academies Press (US).

Kachalia, A., Gandhi, T. K., Puopolo, A. L., Yoon, C., Thomas, E. J., Griffey, R., Brennan, T. A., & Studdert, D. M. (2007). Missed and delayed diagnoses in the emergency department: A study of closed malpractice claims from 4 liability insurers. *Annals of Emergency Medicine, 49*, 196–205.

Khalaila, R., Zbidat, W., Anwar, K., Bayya, A., Linton, D. M., & Sviri, S. (2011). Communication difficulties and psychoemotional distress in patients receiving mechanical ventilation. *American Journal of Critical Care, 20*(6), 470–479.

Kress, J. P., Pohlman, A. S., O'Connor, M. F., & Hall, J. B. (2000). Daily interruption of sedative infusions in critically ill patients undergoing mechanical ventilation. *New England Journal of Medicine, 342*(20), 1471–1477.

Law, B. Y., & Chan, E. A. (2015). The experience of learning to speak up: A narrative inquiry on newly graduated registered nurses. *Journal of Clinical Nursing, 24*, 1837–1848.

Leathart, A. J. (1994). Communication and socialization (1); an exploratory study and explanation for nurse-patient communication in an ITU. *Intensive and Critical Care Nursing, 10*, 93–104.

Leonard, M., Graham, S., & Bonacum, D. (2004). The human factor: The critical importance of effective teamwork and communication in providing safe care. *Quality & Safety in Health Care, 13*(1), i85–i90.

Leung, C. C. H., Pun, J., Lock, G., Slade, D., Gomersall, C. D., Wong, W. T., & Joynt, G. M. (2018). Exploring the scope of communication content of mechanically ventilated patients. *Journal of Critical Care, 44*, 136–141.

Lingard, L., Espin, S., Whyte, S., et al. (2004). Communication failures in the operating room: An observational classification of recurrent types and effects. *Quality & Safety in Health Care, 13*, 330–334.

Luong, J., Yoder, M. K., & Canham, D. (2009). Southeast Asian parents raising a child with autism: A qualitative investigation of coping styles. *The Journal of School Nursing, 25*, 222–229.

Lyndon, A., Sexton, J. B., Simpson, K. R., Rosenstein, A., Lee, K. A., & Wachter, R. M. (2012). Predictors of likelihood of speaking up about safety concerns in labour and delivery. *BMJ Quality & Safety, 21*(9), 791–709.

Magnus, V. S., & Turkington, L. (2006). Communication interaction in ICU—patient and staff experiences and perceptions. *Intensive and Critical Care Nursing, 22*(3), 167–180. https://doi.org/10.1016/j.iccn.2005.10.005

Matthiessen, C. M. I. M. (2013). Applying systemic functional linguistics in healthcare contexts. *Text and Talk, 33*, 437–466.

Mehta, N. M., Bechard, L. J., Cahill, N., Wang, M., Day, A., Duggan, C. P., & Heyland, D. K. (2012). Nutritional practices and their relationship to clinical outcomes in critically ill children—an international multicentre cohort study. *Critical Care Medicine, 40*(7), 2204–2211. https://doi.org/10.1097/CCM.0b013e31824e18a8 PubMed

Menzel, L. (1998). Factors related to the emotional responses of intubated patients to being unable to speak. *Heart & Lung, 27*, 245–252.

Morrison, E. W., & Milliken, F. J. (2003). Speaking up, remaining silent: The dynamics of voice and silence in organizations. *Journal of Management Studies, 40*, 1353–1358.

Myhren, H., Toien, K., Ekeberg, O., Karlsson, S., Sandvik, L., & Stokland, O. (2009). Patients' memory and psychological distress after ICU stay compared with expectations of the relatives. *Intensive and Critical Care Nursing, 35*(12), 2078–2086.

Ng, G. W. Y., Pun, J. K. H., So, E. H. K., et al. (2017). Speak-up culture in an intensive care unit in Hong Kong: A cross-sectional survey exploring the communication openness perceptions of Chinese doctors and nurses. *BMJ Open, 7*, e015721.

Nolan, T. W. (2000). System changes to improve patient safety. *BMJ, 320*, 771–773.

Patak, L., Gawlinski, A., Fung, N. I., Doering, L., & Berg, J. (2004). Patients' reports of health care practitioner interventions that are related to communication during mechanical ventilation. *Heart & Lung, 33*(5), 308–320.

Patak, L., Gawlinski, A., Fung, N. I., Doering, L., Berg, J., & Henneman, E. A. (2006). Communication boards in critical care: Patients' views. *Applied Nursing Research, 19*(4), 182–190.

Pun, J., Matthiessen, C. M. I. M., Slade, D., & Murray, K. (2015). Factors affecting communication in emergency departments: Doctors and nurses' perceptions of communication in a trilingual ED in Hong Kong. *International Journal of Emergency Medicine, 8*, 48.

Rogers, P. C., Graham, C. R., & Mayes, C. T. (2007). Cultural competence and instructional design: Exploration research into the delivery of online instruction cross-culturally. *Educational Technology Research and Development, 55*, 197–217.

Schwappach, D. L., & Gehring, K. (2014). Trade-offs between voice and silence: A qualitative exploration of oncology staff's decisions to speak up about safety concerns. *BMC Health Services Research, 14*, 303.

Slade, D., Manidis, M., McGregor, J., et al. (2011a). *Communicating in Hospital Emergency Departments: Volume 1: Final Report.* University of Technology Sydney.

Slade, D., Manidis, M., McGregor, J., Scheeres, H., et al. (2011b). *Communicating in Hospital Emergency Departments: Final Report.* University of Technology Sydney.

Slade, D., Chandler, E., Pun, J., et al. (2015a). Effective healthcare worker-patient communication in Hong Kong accident and emergency departments. *Hong Kong Journal of Emergency Medicine, 22*(2), 69–83.

Slade, D., Manidis, M., McGregor, J., et al. (2015b). *Communicating in Hospital Emergency Departments.* Springer.

Slade, D., Pun, J., Lock, G., & Eggins, S. (2016). Potential risk points in doctor-patient communication: An analysis of Hong Kong emergency department medical consultations. In H. D. S. Joyce (Ed.), *Language at Work: Analysing Language Use in Work, Education, Medical and Museum Contexts* (pp. 146–165). Cambridge Scholars Publishing.

Society of Critical Care Medicine. (2001). *ICU Patient Communicator App.* Retrieved from http://www.sccm.org/Education-Center/Clinical-Resources/Pages/Patient-and-Family.aspx

Sutcliffe, K. M., Lewton, E., & Rosenthal, M. N. (2004). Communication failures: An insidious contributor to medical mishaps. *Academic Medicine, 79*, 186–194.

Tembo, A. C., Higgins, I., & Parker, V. (2015). The experience of communication difficulties in critically ill patients in and beyond intensive care: Findings from a larger phenomenological study. *Intensive and Critical Care Nursing, 31*(3), 171–178.

ten Hoorn, S., Elbers, P. W., Girbes, A. R., & Tuinman, P. R. (2016). Communicating with conscious and mechanically ventilated critically ill patients: A systematic review. *Critical Care, 20*(1), 333.

Thompson, J. E., Collett, L. W., Langbart, M. J., Purcell, N. J., Boyd, S. M., Yurninaga, Y., Ossolinski, G., Susanto, C., & McCornack, A. (2011). Using the ISBAR handover tool in junior medical officer handover: A study in an Australian tertiary hospital. *Postgrad Medical Journal, 87*, 340–344.

Timmins, C. L. (2002). The impact of language barriers on the health care of Latinos in the United States: A review of the literature and guidelines for practice. *Journal of Midwifery & Women's Health, 47*, 80–96.

Vasquez, C., & Javier, R. A. (1991). The problem with interpreters: Communicating with Spanish-speaking patients. *Psychiatric Services, 42*, 163–165.

Ye, K., McD Taylor, D., Knott, J. C., Dent, A., & MacBean, C. E. (2007). Handover in the emergency department: Deficiencies and adverse effects. *Emergency Medicine Australasia, 19*, 433–441.

4

Research Clinician-to-Clinician Communication at Handovers

Clinician-to-Clinician Communication at Handovers

Modern hospitals face increasing complexity and accelerated operations, which, coupled with high patient loads, make it harder for clinicians to maintain effective communication with colleagues and patients (Slade et al., 2018a, 2018b). Studies reveal that clinicians face unprecedented pressures (Eggins & Slade, 2015; Pun et al., 2015; Slade et al., 2015). Furthermore, research shows that junior doctors and nurses often avoid voicing concerns about patient risks, even when communication tools are standardized (Schwappach & Gehring, 2014).

To address these issues, clinicians require proper training, institutional support, and standardized policies for effective communication, particularly during patient care transitions (Slade et al., 2018a, 2018b). Creating an environment that encourages open communication, where staff feel safe to share concerns and use critical language, is also essential (Leonard et al., 2004). Despite its importance, many nurses lack sufficient training in clinical communication during handovers and often work in settings that do not promote interactive discussions about patient safety (Cleland

J. Pun, *Exploring and Teaching Healthcare Communication*,
https://doi.org/10.1007/978-3-031-08675-5_4

et al., 2009; Jeffcott et al., 2009). Stressful and hierarchical medical environments further exacerbate communication challenges, highlighting the need for more research into how professional pressures impact communication failures (Eggins et al., 2016).

This chapter examines how nurses exchange medical information during handovers in Hong Kong hospitals and their perceptions of clinician communication. Researchers recorded ten handover sessions in medical and surgical wards and interviewed hospital administrators, nurse managers, and nursing staff. Using ethnographic methods and discourse analysis, the team identified communication patterns and structural elements in handovers. Four key areas for improving patient care and safety emerged:

1. Employing a standardized structure for presenting handover information ensures safety and consistency.
2. Incoming nurses should actively participate by checking, clarifying, and confirming details.
3. Outgoing nurses must explicitly transfer responsibility, confirming key details such as care instructions.
4. Nurses need access to relevant documentation during handovers and training on enhancing verbal communication to complement written records.

These recommendations would also enable staff to adapt to bedside handovers, an increasingly preferred global practice.

From the Angle of Ethnography: Multilingual and Multicultural Communication Challenges Faced by Clinicians and Their Students

To learn about the multilingual and multicultural aspects of clinical communication, the research team collaborated with clinicians, linguists, and experts in clinician communication who had previously studied handover communication through an ethnographic discourse analysis approach.

The study took place in Hong Kong, a city with a trilingual environment where people communicate orally in Cantonese, Mandarin, and English, and write in both traditional Chinese and English, which distinguishes it from other Chinese regions. The clinicians involved were all native Chinese speakers who had received medical education in English. Observations revealed that these clinicians used various languages in their daily hospital routines. Clinicians typically read and record medical data in English, but interacted with patients in spoken Cantonese. In clinician-to-clinician communication, they conversed in Cantonese, often mixing in medical English terminology.

Given Hong Kong's trilingual setting, clinical handovers become a complex multilingual process. These interactions are often lengthy, challenging to document, and susceptible to errors (Pun et al., 2015). This chapter aims to help medical students understand how clinicians utilize language in specific institutional contexts to convey meaning and achieve professional objectives.

The research team conducted an ethnographic study to observe clinicians in their natural settings, focusing on the cultural interpretations of their handover behaviours (Heath, 1982). By observing nurses and understanding how they organized their actions, the researchers were able to combine ethnography with discourse analysis to deepen their understanding of social behaviours during handovers. This chapter helps medical students apply a systematic approach to analyse and evaluate clinicians' communication behaviours, allowing them to form informed views on clinician-to-clinician interactions (Chandler et al., 2015; Pun et al., 2015, 2016, 2017; Slade et al., 2015; Slade et al., 2016). It also guides students in communicating effectively to facilitate handovers, enhancing patient safety and ensuring continuity of care.

Current Limitations with the ISBAR Protocol and Its Implementation in Hong Kong

The ISBAR (Identify, Situation, Background, Assessment and Recommendation) protocol is widely recognized as a key tool for guiding structured handover communication globally. It has been extensively adopted to help clinicians organize information effectively during handovers (Pun, 2021). In Hong Kong, the Hospital Authority (HA) has endorsed ISBAR as the primary framework used by frontline clinicians (Hui, 2016). The hospital featured in this study also relied on this protocol. However, despite HA's efforts to standardize communication practices, researchers have observed significant variations in the way nursing handovers are conducted in local hospitals, including the one analysed in this chapter (Ko et al., 2019). Some nurses adhered to a logical sequence when presenting information, while others preferred a more narrative and descriptive style (Pun, 2021).

These inconsistencies in communication have been shown to pose risks to patient safety. Eggins et al. (2016) highlighted how poorly structured or incomplete handover information can lead to confusion or ambiguity. This issue is often exacerbated by the fast-paced clinical environment, which leaves nurses with little time to interact or clarify details during handovers (Pun, 2021). Furthermore, hierarchical workplace dynamics often discourage nurses from voicing their concerns or opinions during these transitions (Omura et al., 2018; Brunton & Cook, 2018). As a result, even when handover information is unclear, nurses may not seek clarification or raise questions (Ginsburg, 2015; Vretare & Anderzen-Carlsson, 2020).

In addition, some studies have pointed out limitations in standardized tools like ISBAR. Giske et al. (2018), Spooner et al. (2016), and Methangkool et al. (2019) noted that checklists do not always guarantee consistency in handover practices, even among experienced nurses. For example, while ISBAR may prompt more frequent questions about ambiguous information, errors can still occur, and the perceived quality of handovers may remain low (Slade et al., 2018a, 2018b). Eggins et al. (2016) further argued that nurses' limited understanding of handover communication reduces the effectiveness of ISBAR in improving communication skills during transitions.

Previous research indicates that the quality of handovers depends not only on the use of standardized tools but also on nurses' communication abilities and their interpretation of these frameworks. Anderson et al. (2015) noted a lack of comprehensive studies on optimizing handover practices. Consequently, the goal of this study was to identify factors influencing nurses' perceptions of handover quality and propose a model illustrating how these factors interact (Pun, 2021).

Testing the Effectiveness of the Revised Protocols

Through analysing audio recordings of observed handovers, researchers highlighted traits of both successful and flawed communication. They specifically pinpointed moments of breakdowns and critical vulnerabilities that could compromise patient safety or the quality of care. These insights allowed nursing students and researchers to examine how outgoing nurses initiated, responded, and followed up with incoming colleagues.

The analysis also explored the use of various communication practices and discourse strategies for transferring patient information. This included examining openness versus closedness, question types, turn-taking, and pauses. From the collected data, researchers observed that participants generally conveyed medical information in a professional and efficient manner.

By reviewing the audio and video recordings, the team identified three key strategies to maintain patient safety and care continuity (See more Eggins et al, 2016):

1. Outgoing nurses should explicitly hand over their responsibilities to incoming colleagues.
2. Incoming nurses must actively participate during handovers.
3. All nursing staff should adhere to a structured handover framework.

The following sections delve deeper into these three themes, shedding light on nurses' perspectives regarding their clinical handover practices.

Instructing Outgoing Nurses to Transfer Responsibilities Clearly

During training, researchers guided nurses in using a revised ISBAR-based worksheet for transferring medical information. Participants were also encouraged to complement this worksheet with verbal handovers structured according to the staged ISBAR framework. By adhering to these procedures, nurses ensured that all ISBAR stages were addressed, making the handover process more logical and predictable. The transfer of information followed a clear "past–present–future" trajectory.

This approach enabled nurses to organize and communicate medical information in distinct sections aligned with the ISBAR structure. Staging markers were introduced to signal transitions between stages, helping to clarify the progression. For instance, an outgoing nurse effectively presented the sequence of Identification (I), Situation (S), and Background (B) in the following Excerpt 1:

Extract 1

Outgoing Nurse:

(ISB): Then, ten-one-three-one, a case newly admitted yesterday. Her doctors are Dr. XYZ and Dr. LMN.

(ISB): She is a 59-year-old lady who has CA of the left brain, with brain secondary. She visited ZZ Hospital in 2016. She was diagnosed with CA of the breast. It was not followed up until April 2018, when her response began to slow. Then, there was some leakage of fluid on the left breast. *[Nurse: nods].* Therefore, she consulted Dr. XYZ. She was admitted for an examination. *[Nurse: nods].*

(ISB): She is allergic to plaster. Good past health. In 2015, she once visited WW Hospital because of a bone fracture, and a left foot surgery was performed in WW Hospital.

Following the completion of their training sessions, researchers observed that outgoing nurses were able to clearly transfer responsibilities by confirming essential details with their colleagues. For example, in Extract 2, one outgoing nurse reiterated the shared information and verified with an incoming colleague whether they fully understood and accepted the instructions regarding the patient's wound care:

Extract 2

Nurse 5 (Outgoing): Yes, she is fasting for her CT. *[N6 nods].* For a guided lung biopsy. **Please do this. Okay?** ***[to N3].*** **Please do it.**
Nurse 3 (Incoming): Yes. *[Nodding]*
Nurse 6 (Outgoing): Any questions? *[to N3]*
Nurse 5 (Outgoing): **Is it okay about the dressing?**
Nurse 2 (Incoming): Yes. *[Nodding]*

In below Extract 3, an outgoing nurse similarly provided a detailed explanation of the tasks required for the afternoon shift. Additionally, she ensured clarity by verifying the incoming nurses' comprehension:

Extract 3

N (Outgoing): Yes, *[N(HO) points at N5's document].* **For you, PM shift, see when Dr. XYZ will inform you to do ECG and ECHO.**
N2 (Incoming): It was just ordered today?
N (Outgoing): This just happened. Wait for him to inform. *[N(HO) flipping her own document].* There is nothing special. He said he will bring this along by himself. He will be discharged tomorrow. So, you should see when he is free.

During training, the team encouraged nurses to demonstrate the ISBAR structure of their clinical handovers using staging markers like "next," "then," "now," and "turning to." Observations revealed that trained participants adopted this approach following the sessions. Evidence of this can be seen in Extract 4 below, where the outgoing nurse presented the Identification, Situation, and Background stages in a clear, sequential manner and used a framing phrase—translated as "then" in English—to transition to the Actions/Assessment stage:

Extract 4

N (Outgoing): This is ten-one-four-five, Dr. XYZ's patient. Has NPC, mucositis. Because of undergoing RT electrotherapy, the neck and mouth are affected. Therefore, he cannot eat. *[N nods].* He was admitted to receive an injection with TPN and continue with RT. That's why he was admitted.

N (Incoming): Um.

N (Outgoing): Then, he is stable. His appetite continues to be poor. For an oral ulcer *[N5 nods],* Dynastat is being injected for pain relief. It's IVI. The headache is still uncomfortable for him, um, around two points on the scale. He once before had nausea. *[N nods].* Therefore, there is a Zofran prn injection for him.

The researchers helped participants interpret the "R" in ISBAR in two ways, namely "Recommendations" and "Readback." These interpretations emphasized the responsibilities of outgoing nurses during the final handover stage, which included: (1) Providing clear instructions for incoming colleagues to follow during their shift and (2) confirming that the information and instructions were clearly understood and acknowledged by the incoming nurses.

Post-training observations showed that participants effectively applied both Recommendations and Readback. For example, in Extract 5 below, the outgoing nurse informed the incoming colleague about actions already taken to dress a patient's wound. Following this, the outgoing nurse repeatedly instructed the incoming nurse to redress the wound.

Extract 5

N (Outgoing): ... There is a wound on the left breast. There is occasional leakage of fluid. The amount is small, pain score is around a point or two. Dr. XYZ once came to visit her yesterday.

N5 (Incoming): Um.

N (Outgoing): To help her dress the wound. It is being covered by Bactigras and pack. Because the left breast ultrasound was done today, *[N5 nods],* the dressing was once removed around the X-ray area. **So, for PM shift, please = =**

N5 (Incoming): = = okay.

N (Outgoing): **Do the dressing one more time.** Already asked Dr. LMN to continue.

To revaluate how effective the updated version of the ISBAR protocol was, the research team reviewed the participants' perceptions of the training sessions' impacts on handover practices:

> *Previously, during handovers, nurses would highlight what they personally considered important rather than presenting a structured, detailed, and complete overview. Looking back, I realize that I may have overlooked some critical points. However, after attending the workshop and adhering to the provided guidelines, reporting information systematically and step-by-step has significantly improved the comprehensiveness of handovers.*
>
> *The ISBAR framework was the most crucial aspect of the workshop, with the information-sharing component being particularly essential. Another key takeaway was the introduction of the handover sheet, which allows nurses to systematically document their work and follow-ups, replacing the use of blank paper.*

Encouraging Active Engagement of Incoming Nurses: The Application of the CARE Model

Before undergoing training, researchers noted that many incoming nurses tended to remain passive during handovers. They rarely sought clarification, even when the information provided was vague, incomplete, or inaccurate. However, post-training transcripts showed a significant improvement, as incoming nurses began to engage more actively in the handover process. They initiated a greater number of questions and verification checks, as seen in Extracts 6 and 7.

Although nurses in medical wards exhibited a higher frequency of interaction compared to their counterparts in surgical wards, all participants demonstrated substantial changes in their communication practices after training. The researchers observed that incoming nurses became more inclined to seek clarification from outgoing colleagues when faced with unclear information. Extracts from clinical handovers illustrated various examples of how incoming nurses participate more actively, and researchers noted that outgoing nurses responded promptly to these queries.

Extract 6

N (Outgoing): She is allergic to plaster. Good past health. In 2016, she once visited ZZ Hospital because of a bone... because of a bone fracture, and a left foot surgery was performed in ZZ Hospital.

N5 (Incoming): **Can she walk?**

N: She can, okay. But her response is rather slow.

N5: Um. *[N5 nods].*

Extract 7

N (Outgoing): Do the dressing one more time. Already asked Dr. XYZ to continue.

N6 (Incoming): For this patient, was the wound already there yesterday?

N (Outgoing): Yes, there is a wound.

N5 (Incoming): Has the skin broken down? Any signs of erosion or ulceration?

N (Outgoing): It is already = = skin broken down. Skin erosion/ulceration.

In Extract 8 below, the incoming staff reiterated the instructions provided by the outgoing nurses to confirm their accurate understanding of the shared information. During this process, N4 sought clarification regarding the guidance offered earlier in the handover:

Extract 8

N(HO): *[Checks the progress sheet, pointing to the physician's orders to N2 and N3]* Here, X-ray. *[N2 + N3 look at the progress sheet]* It was ordered yesterday and completed today. *[N2 nods]* There's another plan; he could have his clips removed on 12th September, which is Wednesday. *[N2 nods head] (Dr. XYZ will assist him.)*

N2: *(Dr. XYZ will assist him.)*

N(HO): Then, planning for discharge.

N5: So, **there are two things to complete.**

N(HO): Yes.

N5: OK.

The evaluations revealed a significant increase in incoming nurses' participation during handovers, as evidenced by the frequency of self-checks. Through these self-checks, the incoming staff verified their understanding of all shared information, ensuring no additional clarification was needed from the outgoing nurses. For instance, in Extract 9 below, one incoming nurse (N3) validated the details with another (N2), after which the outgoing nurse further reviewed the information with both N3 and N2:

Extract 9

N(HO): *(He usually urinated twice in one shift.)*
N2: He usually has a large amount of urine?
N(HO): Yes. *(Pause)*
N2: Anything else?
N(HO): Yes, so let's see when the physiotherapist will come tonight. *(To N2)* His physiotherapy usually starts at 5 PM. *[N2 looks at N(HO)]*
N3: OK.
N(HO): Let's check today's arrangement.
N3: So, we still have the bath not yet completed.
N2: OK.
N3: **Yes, we need to wait to notify his wife about his bath. Then we need to help him.**
N(HO): So, there's nothing else for this case.

A comparable communication pattern was observed in Extract 10, where the incoming nurses requested confirmation from the outgoing nurse to ensure the handover process (turn 146) was fully completed. This made the conclusion of the handover in Extract 10 more collaborative and interactive compared to pre-training practices:

Extract 10

137 N(HO): *(He usually urinates twice in one shift.)*
138 N3: He usually has a large amount of urine?
139 N(HO): Yes. *(Pause)*
140 N3: Anything else?
141 N(HO): Yes, so let's check when the physiotherapist will come tonight. *(To N3)* His physiotherapy usually starts at 5 PM. *[N3 looks at N(HO)]*
142 N4: OK.
143 N(HO): Let's go over today's arrangement.
144 N4: So, we still have the bath not yet completed.
145 N3: OK.
146 N4: **Yes, we need to wait to notify his wife about his bath. Then we need to assist him.**
147 N(HO): So, there's nothing else for this case.

In summary, training incoming nurses to actively engage in exchanges led to faster information sharing through efficient handling of questions. Unlike pre-training scenarios, participants completed handovers more quickly, potentially enhancing patient safety.

Outgoing Nurses' Implementation of CARE

Prior to training, outgoing nurses rarely confirmed whether the information they shared was received and understood by their incoming counterparts. They also seldom encouraged their colleagues to ask questions during handovers. However, video recordings and transcripts revealed a noticeable change in the communication practices of outgoing nurses after the training sessions. They began routinely concluding handovers by inviting their incoming colleagues to ask questions.

For instance, in the above extracts, the outgoing nurse wrapped up the handover by verifying that the incoming staff had no additional questions. Additionally, she reiterated the tasks that needed to be completed by the incoming team:

> *Using the ISBAR framework reduces the time spent on writing, while the CARE protocol encourages more interaction during handovers, making communication more efficient.*
>
> *The introduction of ISBAR and CARE in the workshop has been highly beneficial. These frameworks enhance nurses' communication skills, emphasize the importance of providing feedback, and promote greater interaction and eye contact during handovers. The workshop also helped us recognize our own areas for improvement. After attending, handovers became more structured and time-efficient. Additionally, we gained practical insights on applying these concepts, which has helped us guide junior staff in conducting proper handovers.*

Increased Nurses' Compliance to a New Systematic Handover Structure: Improvements in Communication Between Incoming and Outgoing Colleagues

As previously mentioned, the researchers identified the absence of a consistent structure in nursing handovers. This issue could result in critical information being overlooked, as outgoing nurses might forget details, and incoming staff might fail to notice such omissions. To resolve this problem, the team developed an updated worksheet by adapting the ISBAR framework. Post-training videos revealed that all participants utilized the revised structure to both present and request information. The team observed that, after training, the handovers followed a more organized sequence, enabling incoming nurses to seek clarification on planned assessments and treatment strategies for their patients (see Extract 11).

Extract 11

N(HO): Yes, she is fasting for her CT. *[N4 nods]*. For a guided lung biopsy. Please do this. Okay? *[to N3]*. Please do it.

N4: Any questions? *[to N3]*

N(HO): Is everything okay with the dressing?

The participating nurses elaborated on how the revised ISBAR worksheet made handovers more effective:

> *Following the training, the ward sheet has been a useful guide for nurses, helping them structure their thought process and ensuring a smooth handover. The handovers have become more organized, making communication clearer and more effective than before.*
>
> *The grid layout in the ward sheet is particularly helpful, providing a practical reference for nurses during handovers. Compared to the posters, which were seen as less effective, the ward sheet offers a more hands-on approach. It keeps nurses more attentive to key details, reducing the likelihood of missing important information.*

As per the nurses in these interviews, the revised model helped them in organizing thoughts systematically and preventing them from missing key information during handover processes.

Nurses' Perceptions of the CARE Protocol and Patient-Centred Communication

The study's findings highlight the value of using the CARE protocol (Connect, Ask, Readback, and Engage) during handovers. By applying it, nursing staff were able to facilitate effective communication through interactive exchanges, collaborative efforts, and a focus on patient-centred care. Post-training, nurses demonstrated more active engagement, as the training helped them thoroughly understand the principles underlying patient-centred clinical handovers. This improvement enabled them to communicate more clearly and lead structured, interactive handover processes.

In Hong Kong's bilingual clinical environment, nurses who adhered to the CARE protocol showed improved focus, allowing them to engage in more meaningful and effective communication with both patients and colleagues. Additionally, the participants developed a heightened appreciation for the importance of handover communication, recognizing its impact on patient safety and continuity of care (Pun et al., 2018). This shift in perspective marked a significant advancement in local clinical communication practices, especially given the delays in the Hospital Authority's formal implementation of patient-centred care as an official policy (Hospital Authority, 2018).

The participating nurses highlighted significant advantages of training both nursing students and practicing nurses using a structured, interactive, and patient-centred handover protocol, as demonstrated in the above extracts. They emphasized that such training helps them provide "a clear, systematic, and comprehensive picture" when sharing medical information with colleagues. Consequently, medical educators are strongly encouraged to teach students structured protocols to aid in identifying, sharing, discussing, and confirming critical informational and interpersonal aspects of patient-centred care. Beyond opportunities to ask questions and perceptions of the ISBAR protocol, the study uncovered other factors that contribute to improved handover quality, which can serve as valuable teaching references in medical education. Additionally, nursing students should recognize that asking questions and obtaining updated information during handovers enhances their understanding of patient care plans. The training programme described in the study acted as an effective educational tool, guiding nurses "through the processes and thinking and helped them to follow through with the handover smoothly" within a structured framework, as noted by interviewees. This approach enables students to gather and document both medical and social or personal information in a more organized manner (Pun et al., 2018). Ultimately, this should equip future nurses with the skills to gain a thorough and accurate understanding of their patients' medical histories, conditions, and prognoses.

To assess the impact of the training sessions, the researchers compared the quality of clinical handovers conducted by nurses before and after training. The evaluations focused on the exchange of patient information under the ISBAR framework and interaction levels based on the CARE-team protocol. The findings revealed notable improvements. For instance, participants demonstrated better emotional expression, conveyed information more effectively, enhanced teamwork, and conducted handovers in a more organized manner. However, the training did not significantly increase the level of interaction during handovers, as scores for this aspect remained relatively unchanged. Literature on professional training emphasizes that successful outcomes often rely on consistent, long-term support from organizations (Chisengantambu et al., 2018). Therefore, local hospitals need to implement continuous, sustained efforts to reinforce newly introduced practices beyond the initial training phase.

The study findings suggest that future research should aim to refine and develop handover protocols to teach nursing students systematic approaches to exchanging medical information. This is particularly important for improving communication among incoming nurses, patients, and caregivers (Pun et al., 2020). While many studies focus on the role of outgoing nurses in sharing information (Holly & Poletick, 2014), it is equally important for hospitals to encourage collaboration among all stakeholders during handovers, as this impacts patient care quality. Disseminating protocols like ISBAR (Bakon et al., 2017; Thomson et al., 2018) and emphasizing the importance of interactions under the CARE protocol (Eggins & Slade, 2015; Slade et al., 2018a, 2018b) can enhance communication practices.

To improve educational tools for medical schools and nursing programmes, researchers should continue testing the CARE protocol's effectiveness across diverse clinical settings, including different types of wards and bedside handovers involving patients (Redley & Waugh, 2018). Developing standardized approaches to nursing handovers, such as the CARE protocol, could encourage teamwork, interactive communication, and patient-centred care (Pun et al., 2020). Nonetheless, further evaluations of the revised ISBAR and CARE frameworks are necessary to ensure their effectiveness.

Overall, training programmes for nurses and students can produce substantial short-term benefits and contribute to long-term improvements in patient care if prioritized institutionally (Lee et al., 2012; Manser & Foster, 2011; De Meester et al., 2013). Continuous communication training provided by medical schools and hospitals could reduce the frequency and severity of critical incidents, enhance interdisciplinary collaboration, promote patient-centred practices, and improve staff retention (Bakon et al., 2017; Eggins & Slade, 2015).

Limitations of the Study

Given the limited sample size—ten audio and video recordings documenting handovers across 80 patient cases at a single hospital—the study's findings may include some biases. However, the collected recordings and transcripts still provided valuable insights into existing communication challenges during handovers and highlighted the potential benefits of targeted training using the revised ISBAR and CARE protocols. Additionally, the study offered nursing students a deeper understanding of the unique characteristics of clinical settings in Hong Kong.

* * *

Analysis of the data and performance evaluations from pre- and post-training handovers showed that the revised ISBAR worksheet and CARE protocol significantly enhanced communication effectiveness. A notable change was observed in nurses' handover practices: prior to training, handovers were largely monologic, with incoming staff displaying a passive role. Post-training, handovers became more collaborative, with participants showing active engagement in comprehending patient cases. The newly designed ISBAR protocol proved to be an effective framework for organizing and delivering structured nursing handovers. Thus, medical educators are encouraged to incorporate similar training programmes to emphasize the importance of handover communication and the shared responsibility of providing patient-centred care.

The study also highlighted the value of employing an ethnographic discourse analysis approach. This interdisciplinary method allowed researchers to identify key features of both effective and ineffective communication within local nursing contexts. It provided a robust foundation for assessing the impact of newly designed training programmes, ultimately contributing to improved professional handover practices. Future researchers are encouraged to adopt this methodology when examining the complex dimensions of discourse and social interactions in their chosen cultural settings. This approach could offer a more nuanced understanding of communication dynamics and inform the development of tailored solutions.

References

Anderson, J., Malone, L., Shanahan, K., & Manning, J. (2015). Nursing bedside clinical handover—An integrated review of issues and tools. *Journal of Clinical Nursing, 24*(5–6), 662–671.

Bakon, S., Wirihana, L., Christensen, M., & Craft, J. (2017). Nursing handovers: An integrative review of the different models and processes available. *International Journal of Nursing Practice, 23*(2), e12520.

Brunton, M., & Cook, C. (2018). Dis/integrating cultural difference in practice and communication: A qualitative study of host and migrant registered nurse perspectives from New Zealand. *International Journal of Nursing Studies, 83*, 18–24.

Chandler, E., Slade, D., Pun, J., Espindola, E., Lock, G., Matthiessen, C. M. I. M., & Ng, C. (2015). Communication in Hong Kong Accident & Emergency Departments: The clinicians' perspective. *Global Qualitative Nursing Research, 2*, 1–11.

Chisengantambu, C., Robinson, G. M., & Evans, N. (2018). Nurse managers and the sandwich support model. *Journal of Nursing Management, 26*, 192–199.

Cleland, J. A., Ross, S., Miller, S. C., & Patey, R. (2009). "There is a chain of Chinese whispers…": Empirical data support the call to formally teach handover to prequalification doctors. *BMJ Quality & Safety, 18*(4), 267–271.

De Meester, K., Verspuy, M., Monsieurs, K. G., & Van Bogaert, P. (2013). SBAR improves nurse–physician communication and reduces unexpected death: A pre and post intervention study. *Resuscitation, 84*(9), 1192–1196.

Eggins, S., & Slade, D. (2015). Communication in clinical handover: Improving the safety and quality of the patient experience. *Journal of Public Health Research, 4*(3), 666.

Eggins, S., Slade, D., & Geddes, F. (Eds.). (2016). *Effective communication in clinical handover—From research to practice*. De Gruyter Mouton.

Ginsburg, L. (2015). 'Speaking up' climate: A new domain of culture to measure and explore. *BMJ Quality & Safety, 24*, 661–663.

Giske, T., Melås, S. N., & Einarsen, K. A. (2018). The art of oral handovers: A participant observational study by undergraduate students in a hospital setting. *Journal of Clinical Nursing, 27*(5–6), e767–e775.

Heath, S. B. (1982). Ethnography in education: Defining the essentials. In P. Gilmore & A. A. Glatthorn (Eds.), *Children in and out of school: Ethnography and education* (pp. 33–58). Center for Applied Linguistics.

Holly, C., & Poletick, E. B. (2014). A systematic review on the transfer of information during nurse transitions in care. *Journal of Clinical Nursing, 23*, 2387–2396.

Hospital Authority (HA). (2018). *Quality Times* (23). Retrieved from https://www.ha.org.hk/haho/ho/qs/Quality_Times_Issue_23_en.pdf

Hui, J. (2016). I-PASS. The hospital authority periodic publication on quality improvement for healthcare professionals. *Quality Times, 23*(1).

Jeffcott, S. A., Ibrahim, J. E., & Cameron, P. A. (2009). Resilience in health-care and clinical handover. *BMJ Quality and Safety, 18*(4), 256–260.

Ko, Y. T. P., Tse, K. M., Yeung, M. F., Chan, L. P., Woo, M. C., & Tang, S. W. (2019). Effective clinical handover enhances better communication and patient safety across multidisciplinary healthcare professions in a rehabilitation hospital. *Hospital Authority*.

Lee, P., Allen, K., & Daly, M. A. (2012). Communication and Patient Safety training programme for all healthcare staff: Can it make a difference? *BMJ Quality and Safety, 21*, 84–88.

Leonard, M., Graham, S., & Bonacum, D. (2004). The human factor: The critical importance of effective teamwork and communication in providing safe care. *Quality and Safety in Health Care, 13*(Suppl. 1), 85–90.

Manser, T., & Foster, S. (2011). Effective handover communication: An overview of research and improvement efforts. *Best Practice & Research Clinical Anaesthesiology, 25*, 181–191.

Methangkool, E., Tollinche, L., Sparling, J., & Agarwala, A. V. (2019). Communication: Is there a standard handover technique to transfer patient care? *International Anesthesiology Clinics, 57*(3), 35–47.

Omura, M., Stone, T. E., & Levett-Jones, T. (2018). Cultural factors influencing Japanese nurses' assertive communication. Part 1: Collectivism. *Nursing & Health Sciences, 20*(3), 283–288.

Pun, J. (2021). Factors associated with nurses' perceptions, their communication skills and the quality of clinical handover in the Hong Kong context. *BCM Nursing, 20*, 95.

Pun, J., Matthiessen, C. M. I. M., Slade, D., & Murray, K. (2015). Factors affecting communication in emergency departments: Doctors and nurses' perceptions of communication in a trilingual ED in Hong Kong. *International Journal of Emergency Medicine, 8*, 48.

Pun, J., Chan, E. A., Murray, K. A., Slade, D., & Matthiessen, C. M. I. M. (2016). Clinicians' perceptions of communication challenges in a trilingual emergency department in Hong Kong. *Journal of Clinical Nursing, 26*, 3396–3407.

Pun, J., Matthiessen, C. M. I. M., Williams, G., & Slade, D. (2017). Using ethnographic discourse analysis to understand doctor-patient interactions in clinical settings. *SAGE Research Methods Cases*.

Pun, J., Chan, E. A., Man, M., Eggins, S., & Slade, D. (2018). Pre- and post evaluations of the effects of the Connect, Ask, Respond and Empathise (CARE) protocol on nursing handover: A case study of a bilingual hospital in Hong Kong. *Journal of Clinical Nursing, 28*, 3001–3011.

Pun, J., Chan, E. A., Eggins, S., & Slade, D. (2020). Training in communication and interaction during shift-to-shift nursing handovers in a bilingual hospital: A case study. *Nurse Education Today, 84*, e104212.

Redley, B., & Waugh, R. (2018). Mixed methods evaluation of a quality improvement and audit tool for nurse-to-nurse bedside clinical handover in ward settings. *Applied Nursing Research, 40*, 80–89.

Schwappach, D. L., & Gehring, K. (2014). Trade-offs between voice and silence: A qualitative exploration of oncology staff's decisions to speak up about safety concerns. *BMC Health Services Research, 14*(1), 303.

Slade, D., Chandler, E., Pun, J., Lam, M., et al. (2015). Effective healthcare worker-patient communication in Hong Kong accident and emergency departments. *Hong Kong Journal of Emergency Medicine, 22*(2), 69–83.

Slade, D., Murray, K. A., Pun, J. K. H., & Eggins, S. (2018a). Nurses' perceptions of mandatory bedside clinical handovers: An Australian hospital study. *Journal of Nursing Management, 27*, 161–171.

Slade, D., Pun, J., & Lock, G. (2016). Potential Risk Points in Doctor–Patient Communication: An Analysis of Hong Kong Emergency Department Medical Consultations. In H. de Silva Joyce (Ed.), *Language at Work: Analysing Language Use in Work, Education, Medical and Museum Contexts* (pp. 146–165). Cambridge Scholars Publishing.

Slade, D., Pun, J., Murray, K. A., & Eggins, S. (2018b). Benefits of health care communication training for nurses conducting bedside handovers: An Australian hospital case study. *Journal of Continuing Education in Nursing, 49*(7), 329–336.

Spooner, A. J., Aitken, L. M., Corley, A., Fraser, J. F., & Chaboyer, W. (2016). Nursing team leader handover in the intensive care unit contains diverse and inconsistent content: An observational study. *International Journal of Nursing Studies, 61*, 165–172.

Thomson, H., Tourangeau, A., Jeffs, L., & Puts, M. (2018). Factors affecting quality of nurse shift handover in the emergency department. *Journal of Advanced Nursing, 74*, 876–886.

Vretare, L. L., & Anderzen-Carlsson, A. (2020). The critical care nurse's perception of handover: A phenomenographic study. *Intensive & Critical Care Nursing, 58*, 102807.

5

Understanding High-Risk Multilingual Communication in Accident & Emergency Departments (AEDs)

Navigating Multilingual Communication Challenges in High-Pressure AED Settings

Accident and Emergency Departments (AEDs) are high-pressure environments where effective communication plays a critical role in ensuring patient safety and care quality. In Hong Kong's trilingual clinical context—where Cantonese, Mandarin, and English intersect—communication challenges are magnified, posing unique risks to healthcare outcomes. This chapter explores the complexity of multilingual communication in AEDs, examines patient participation in shared decision-making, and identifies strategies to mitigate risks in this setting.

Effective clinical communication is essential for delivering high-quality healthcare services, particularly in high-risk, time-pressured environments such as accident & emergency departments (AEDs) (Slade et al., 2011a, 2011b). Communication challenges in EDs are especially pronounced in multilingual contexts like Hong Kong. For instance, Slade et al. (2015a, 2015b) identified several communication issues in Hong Kong's accident and emergency departments (AEDs): (1) clinicians struggled to establish rapport and demonstrate empathy due to stress and

J. Pun, *Exploring and Teaching Healthcare Communication*,
https://doi.org/10.1007/978-3-031-08675-5_5

time constraints; (2) healthcare workers frequently misinterpreted verbal information during interactions; (3) handovers between senior and junior staff were often ineffective; (4) patient information recording was inconsistent, leading to gaps during handovers; and (5) translation processes often distorted or omitted critical patient information. These challenges contribute to inadequate information sharing and unsystematic documentation processes, resulting in adverse patient outcomes such as misdiagnoses, prolonged hospital stays, and missed follow-up appointments (Stiell et al., 2003).

The Trilingual Context of Clinical Communication

Similar to EDs in other Asian and European regions, Hong Kong's AEDs operate in a trilingual environment where Cantonese, Mandarin, and English are commonly used. Clinicians, whose native language is often Chinese, navigate bilingual or trilingual communication during daily tasks. This linguistic dynamic reflects Hong Kong's official language policies and the use of English in tertiary education (Chandler et al., 2015). In practice, clinicians read and document medical information predominantly in English while communicating with patients in their native languages. Among themselves, they primarily converse in Cantonese, often interspersed with English medical terminology (Slade et al., 2015a, 2015b). This blending of languages can lead to inconsistencies in medical documentation. Consequently, translation processes frequently occur throughout a single patient's journey (Matthiessen, 2013). Additionally, clinicians' code-switching can confuse patients, making it challenging for them to comprehend all languages used by their healthcare providers (Slade et al., 2016a, 2016b) (see Fig. 3.1). Thus, this linguistic interplay, coupled with time-sensitive decisions, introduces significant risks for miscommunication and errors (Pun et al., 2015) Interview data reveal that the trilingual context poses unique challenges. For instance, clinicians frequently translate medical information between languages, often leading to omissions or inaccuracies. Such errors are particularly evident during handovers, where spoken instructions in Cantonese or Mandarin may conflict with written English notes. A senior AED doctor noted: "*Sometimes the doctors give verbal instructions, but these are not well understood by the nurses, leading to errors in medication dosage or infusion rates.*"

To mitigate these challenges, some clinicians adopt practices such as incorporating Chinese characters into English notes to preserve meaning during translation. However, the inconsistency in these adaptations underscores the need for systemic strategies to improve multilingual communication. While these adaptive strategies—such as integrating Chinese characters into English notes—help address immediate communication challenges, they reveal deeper systemic issues requiring robust and standardized approaches. This interplay between language and context underscores the critical need for frameworks that prioritize clarity, accuracy, and inclusivity in multilingual healthcare settings. These challenges become even more pronounced when considering the dynamics of shared decision-making (SDM), where effective communication is pivotal in fostering collaboration between clinicians and patients.

Shared Decision-Making in AED Visits

Shared decision-making (SDM) is a collaborative process in which clinicians and patients engage in meaningful discussions to explore treatment options, weigh the potential benefits and risks, and agree on a care plan. This approach is fundamental to patient-centred care, as it respects patients' autonomy and involves them in decisions about their health. However, in the high-pressure, multilingual context of Hong Kong's AEDs, SDM is often constrained by several factors, including language barriers, time limitations, and cultural differences.

Language barriers are a significant obstacle in SDM, as clinicians and patients may not share a common language or struggle with technical terminology. The urgency of AED contexts exacerbates these issues, leaving little time for detailed discussions or clarifications. Additionally, cultural expectations in Hong Kong often position clinicians as authority figures, which can discourage patients from voicing their opinions or preferences during consultations.

Patient interviews reveal that effective SDM is rare in Hong Kong's AEDs, with many patients perceiving consultations as clinician-led. Despite this, linguistic evidence from recorded interactions highlights moments where patients actively participate in decision-making. These include:

1. **Clarifying Symptoms:** Patients often provide detailed descriptions of their conditions, which prompt clinicians to reconsider initial diagnoses or adjust treatment plans. For example, a patient's description of worsening dizziness led a doctor to revise the treatment approach, demonstrating how patient input can influence clinical decisions.
2. **Expressing Preferences:** Patients articulate their preferences regarding specific procedures or medications. These expressions often stem from prior experiences or concerns about side effects, illustrating their role in shaping care plans.
3. **Seeking Reassurance:** Patients frequently ask questions to confirm their understanding of their conditions and treatment options. This dialogue not only builds trust but also ensures that patients are informed participants in their care.

From the clinicians' perspective, balancing patient involvement with the fast-paced demands of AEDs is a persistent challenge. Clinicians emphasize the importance of using clear, jargon-free language to facilitate understanding and creating opportunities for patients to share their perspectives, even within time-constrained scenarios. Simple strategies, such as summarizing key points or using visual aids, can make complex medical information more accessible to patients.

Despite these efforts, the time pressures and hierarchical culture in AEDs often limit the depth of SDM. Many clinicians feel that prioritizing patient involvement is at odds with the need for rapid decision-making in emergency settings. However, fostering SDM—even in small, incremental ways—can significantly enhance patient satisfaction and safety. By building rapport and encouraging open communication, clinicians can ensure that patients feel heard and valued, ultimately improving the overall quality of care.

Transitioning from the intricacies of SDM to the broader communication dynamics within AEDs, it is evident that the linguistic and systemic factors at play in Hong Kong's healthcare context demand further investigation. Understanding these elements is crucial not only for enhancing SDM but also for addressing communication challenges more broadly. The following section delves into the specific context of Hong Kong's AEDs, focusing on the interplay between language, culture, and systemic pressures that shape clinical interactions and outcomes.

The AED Communication in Hong Kong

Given the unique linguistic context and communication challenges in Hong Kong's AEDs, this chapter highlights a study conducted by Pun et al. (2016) that examined communication dynamics between doctors and patients in a local ED. The study offers a detailed analysis of trilingual clinical communication and provides linguistic evidence of patient participation in shared decision-making processes. The research involved 28 interviews with key ED clinicians, audio recordings of 10 patient journeys from triage to disposition, and 58 questionnaires completed by ED clinicians, nurses, and allied healthcare workers. The research team conducted thematic analyses to identify recurring communication issues, thereby establishing a foundation for exploring linguistic evidence relevant to shared decision-making and barriers in trilingual clinical interactions.

The study surveyed 58 clinicians (36 nurses and 22 doctors) and conducted interviews with 28 of them (8 doctors and 20 nurses). Participants had varied lengths of experience in the ED, ranging from 3 months to over 9 years. The chosen ED, one of the busiest in Hong Kong, handles approximately 600 patients daily, with a significant proportion categorized as urgent. Annually, this ED serves over one million patients, representing more than 10% of Hong Kong's population. The research team, comprising seven specialized researchers, conducted the study between August and September 2011. The survey was crafted based on reviews of healthcare communication studies and pilot-tested for clarity and reliability, achieving a Cronbach's alpha of 0.8. Questions covered three key areas: communication processes, medical documentation, and the ED's professional environment. Additionally, audio recordings of ten patient journeys were collected, allowing for an analysis of effective and ineffective clinical interactions.

The study revealed significant communication challenges, including inconsistencies in documentation, time pressures, and frequent miscommunications during handovers and triage. Over 48% of clinicians reported instances of altered information during translations, which often led to errors. Furthermore, clinicians highlighted the difficulties of providing adequate information and engaging in meaningful dialogue with patients in a high-pressure, trilingual environment. These findings underscore the need for improved communication frameworks and tailored strategies to address these systemic issues in Hong Kong's emergency departments. The next section will further review some of these identified communication challenges that are typical to AEDs in Chinese context.

Challenges to Effective Communication in AEDs

Linguistic Barriers

Frequent code-switching between Cantonese, Mandarin, and English complicates accurate information relay. Clinicians face challenges in translating medical terminology on the spot and ensuring that translations are precise and contextually appropriate. Misinterpretations during these translations can lead to misinformation, particularly when dealing with complex medical terms or during high-pressure situations such as handovers and triage.

Time Pressures

High patient volumes and limited clinician availability result in rushed consultations, which often compromise the quality of communication.

Time constraints are particularly critical during triage, where insufficient communication can lead to misclassification of patients, with potentially severe consequences. For instance, a patient incorrectly categorized at triage due to poor communication later suffered significant complications, emphasizing the need for precise and thorough interactions.

Cultural Factors

Hong Kong's hierarchical medical culture discourages junior staff from questioning senior colleagues or voicing concerns, exacerbating communication gaps. Nurses frequently follow doctors' instructions without seeking clarification, while junior doctors may hesitate to challenge decisions made by their senior counterparts. This deference to authority often leads to unaddressed errors or omissions, further compromising patient safety.

Documentation Challenges

Written medical notes are often condensed for efficiency, which compromises the level of detail necessary for effective follow-up care. These brevities, combined with language inconsistencies—such as the frequent use of medical jargon or mixed languages—undermine the continuity of care. Miscommunications during transitions, such as handovers, are amplified when documentation lacks clarity or fails to capture critical patient information comprehensively.

Addressing these barriers requires a combination of systemic changes, cultural shifts, and targeted training. Improved communication frameworks, standardized documentation protocols, and fostering a more open and collaborative workplace culture are essential to overcoming these challenges in Hong Kong's AEDs.

Improving Communication in AEDs

To address these challenges, the chapter proposes a model to enhance healthcare communication from a multilingual perspective. Key recommendations include:

Standardized Communication Protocols

Develop clear guidelines for multilingual communication during handovers to ensure consistency and clarity. Protocols like ISBAR (Introduction, Situation, Background, Assessment, Recommendation) can standardize the flow of information, reducing errors caused by miscommunication. This approach should include multilingual templates for key interactions to accommodate the trilingual environment of Hong Kong AEDs. Regular training sessions on protocol usage should be conducted to reinforce adherence and effectiveness.

Language Training

Provide targeted training programmes to improve clinicians' proficiency in medical Cantonese, Mandarin, and English. These programmes should focus on enhancing vocabulary, refining translation techniques, and building confidence in using medical terminology across languages. Additionally, training should emphasize culturally sensitive communication to ensure that language barriers do not impede patient rapport or care quality. Offering role-play scenarios and case studies can help clinicians practice and apply these skills in real-life settings.

Patient-Centred Practices

Encourage shared decision-making (SDM) by creating dedicated opportunities for patient narratives and clarifications during consultations. Even in high-pressure environments, clinicians should be trained to allocate time for listening to patient concerns, explaining medical procedures in simple terms, and involving patients in treatment decisions. This practice not only improves patient satisfaction but also enhances the accuracy of diagnoses and adherence to treatment plans. Supervisors should monitor and reward clinicians who effectively implement SDM.

Technological Solutions

Leverage digital tools to support accurate and efficient multilingual communication. Multilingual communication apps and real-time translation devices can bridge language gaps and reduce reliance on impromptu translations. These tools should integrate with hospital electronic medical record systems to ensure seamless documentation in the preferred language. Regular updates and staff training on using these technologies can maximize their utility and minimize errors.

Cultural Shifts

Foster a non-hierarchical work culture that empowers all staff members to voice concerns and prioritize patient safety. This can be achieved through psychological safety training, which encourages open dialogue and mutual respect across ranks. Leaders should model inclusive behaviours and create environments where junior staff feel comfortable questioning decisions or seeking clarification. This cultural shift not only improves communication but also reduces risks associated with unchallenged errors.

Conclusion

This chapter has examined the complexities of multilingual communication in Hong Kong's Accident and Emergency Departments (AEDs), highlighting the significant challenges that arise in a trilingual clinical environment where Cantonese, Mandarin, and English are commonly used. Given the critical nature of emergency care, effective communication is essential for ensuring patient safety, delivering high-quality healthcare, and facilitating shared decision-making between clinicians and patients. However, the high-pressure, time-sensitive nature of AEDs, combined with linguistic and cultural factors, creates barriers that hinder effective interactions and may lead to adverse medical outcomes.

The findings of this study reveal that communication difficulties in AEDs manifest in multiple ways. Linguistic challenges, such as frequent code-switching, translation errors, and misunderstandings of medical terminology, complicate clinician-patient interactions. These difficulties are exacerbated by the hierarchical nature of healthcare communication in Hong Kong, where junior staff members may be hesitant to seek clarification or challenge decisions made by senior colleagues, potentially leading to errors in medical documentation and treatment. Additionally, the lack of standardized communication protocols results in inconsistencies in patient handovers, increasing the risk of misdiagnosis, prolonged hospital stays, and improper follow-up care.

Beyond language-related barriers, the study underscores the impact of time constraints on clinical communication. In fast-paced AED settings, consultations are often rushed, leaving limited opportunities for comprehensive patient engagement. As a result, shared decision-making (SDM), a key component of patient-centred care, is frequently compromised. Patients may struggle to fully understand their diagnoses and treatment options, and clinicians may not have the time to facilitate meaningful discussions. The study findings indicate that while some patients actively participate in decision-making—by clarifying symptoms, expressing treatment preferences, or seeking reassurance—these interactions remain sporadic and largely dependent on individual clinician efforts rather than systematic communication practices.

To address these challenges, the chapter proposes a range of strategies aimed at improving multilingual communication and fostering a more inclusive, patient-centred healthcare environment. One of the key recommendations is the adoption of standardized communication protocols, such as ISBAR (Introduction, Situation, Background, Assessment, Recommendation), to ensure consistency and clarity in clinical handovers. Establishing clear linguistic guidelines for clinician-patient interactions can help mitigate the risks associated with ad-hoc translation and code-switching. Additionally, language training programmes tailored to the needs of healthcare professionals in multilingual settings can enhance their ability to navigate trilingual communication effectively. These programmes should focus not only on linguistic proficiency but also on cultural sensitivity and medical terminology across different languages.

The chapter also highlights the potential role of technological innovations in bridging communication gaps. Digital tools, such as real-time translation applications and multilingual electronic health records, can facilitate more accurate and efficient communication, reducing the reliance on impromptu translation by clinicians. However, the effectiveness of such technologies depends on proper implementation, training, and integration with existing hospital systems.

Another critical intervention involves promoting patient-centred communication practices by incorporating structured opportunities for patient engagement. Training healthcare professionals to use simplified, jargon-free language, employ visual aids, and encourage patient participation in medical discussions can significantly improve comprehension and trust. Furthermore, shifting from a hierarchical to a more **collaborative workplace culture**—where junior staff feel empowered to raise concerns and patients are encouraged to voice their preferences—can help mitigate communication breakdowns and enhance overall care quality.

Broader Implications and Future Research Directions

The challenges discussed in this chapter extend beyond Hong Kong and resonate with healthcare systems worldwide that operate in linguistically and culturally diverse environments. The findings contribute to a growing body of research on multilingual healthcare communication, emphasizing the need for institutional policies and structural reforms that facilitate clear, inclusive, and effective clinician-patient interactions.

Future research should focus on assessing the long-term impact of the proposed interventions, particularly in emergency healthcare settings where communication errors can have life-threatening consequences.

Evaluating the effectiveness of standardized protocols, technological solutions, and patient-centred communication training through empirical studies can provide evidence-based recommendations for hospitals and policymakers. Additionally, comparative studies across different multilingual healthcare settings can offer insights into best practices and adaptable strategies that transcend specific cultural and linguistic contexts.

Ultimately, by addressing these systemic communication challenges, healthcare institutions can improve patient outcomes, reduce medical errors, and ensure equitable access to high-quality emergency medical care. As healthcare systems continue to evolve in response to global migration patterns and increasing linguistic diversity, developing robust multilingual communication frameworks will be essential in meeting the needs of diverse patient populations.

References

Chandler, E., Slade, D., Pun, J., Lock, G., Matthiessen, C. M. I. M., Espindola, E., & Ng, C. (2015). Communication in Hong Kong accident & emergency departments: The clinicians' perspectives. *Global Qualitative Nursing Journal, 2*, 1–11.

Matthiessen, C. M. I. M. (2013). Applying systemic functional linguistics in healthcare contexts. *Text and Talk, 33*, 437–466.

Pun, J., Matthiessen, C. M. I. M., Slade, D., & Murray, K. (2015). Factors affecting communication in emergency departments: Doctors and nurses' perceptions of communication in a trilingual ED in Hong Kong. *International Journal of Emergency Medicine, 8*, 48.

Pun, J., Matthiessen, C. M. I. M., Williams, G., & Slade, D. (2016). Using ethnographic discourse analysis to understand doctor-patient interactions in clinical settings. *SAGE Research Methods Case.*

Slade, D., Manidis, M., McGregor, J., Scheeres, H., et al. (2011a). *Communicating in Hospital Emergency Departments: Final Report.* University of Technology Sydney.

Slade, D., Manidis, M., McGregor, J., et al. (2011b). *Communicating in Hospital Emergency Departments: Volume 1: Final Report.* University of Technology Sydney.

Slade, D., Chandler, E., Pun, J., et al. (2015a). Effective healthcare worker-patient communication in Hong Kong accident and emergency departments. *Hong Kong Journal of Emergency Medicine, 22*(2), 69–83.

Slade, D., Manidis, M., McGregor, J., et al. (2015b). *Communicating in Hospital Emergency Departments*. Springer.

Slade, D., Matthiessen, C. M. I. M., Lock, G., Pun, J., & Lam, M. (2016a). The patterns of interaction in doctor-patient communication and their impact on health outcomes. In L. Ortega, A. Tyler, & H. I. Park (Eds.), *The Usage-Based Study of Language Learning and Multilingualism* (pp. 235–254). Georgetown University Press.

Slade, D., Pun, J., Lock, G., & Eggins, S. (2016b). Potential risk points in doctor-patient communication: An analysis of Hong Kong emergency department medical consultations. In H. D. S. Joyce (Ed.), *Language at Work: Analysing Language Use in Work, Education, Medical and Museum Contexts* (pp. 146–165). Cambridge Scholars Publishing.

Stiell, A., Forster, A. J., Stiell, I. G., & van Wal-raven, C. (2003). Prevalence of information gaps in the emergency department and the effect on patient outcomes. *Canadian Medical Association Journal, 169*, 1023–1028.

[illegible]

6

Chinese Clinicians' Perspectives Towards Inter- and Intra-disciplinary Communication Between Staff in the Intensive Care Unit

Why Speak-Up Culture in High-Risk Settings Is Important?

Communication openness, defined by Ayoko (2007) as the ease of verbal interaction and comprehension during conversations, encompasses trust, listening, honesty, and support. Rogers et al. (2007) emphasize that communication openness involves the exchange of messages among peers and hierarchies. Research underscores the critical role of speaking up in enhancing patient safety, mitigating risks associated with poor communication and teamwork failures (Leonard et al., 2004). Speaking up often involves voicing concerns about safety, errors, or omissions, particularly when such issues arise from senior colleagues' actions.

However, studies reveal hesitation among clinicians, particularly junior staff, to voice concerns, often due to hierarchical structures or fear of negative repercussions (Morrison & Milliken, 2003). Factors such as tenure, organizational culture, and training significantly influence clinicians' willingness to speak up. For example, Nembhard et al. (2015) highlighted that organizational contexts and individual attributes shape attitudes toward speaking up. Cultural dimensions also impact this behaviour. In

J. Pun, *Exploring and Teaching Healthcare Communication*,
https://doi.org/10.1007/978-3-031-08675-5_6

Hong Kong, research by Law and Chan (2015) indicated that junior nurses often face generational divides and limited support from senior clinicians, contributing to barriers in raising safety concerns. Studies suggest that fostering communication openness and addressing cultural challenges, particularly in Chinese contexts, is essential to improve safety and teamwork in clinical environments.

Speak-Up Culture in Hong Kong ICU

The concept of speak-up culture encompasses the degree to which clinicians feel secure and empowered to express concerns, pose questions, and offer opinions in high-stakes environments. This culture is critical in Intensive Care Units (ICUs) where timely communication can directly impact patient safety and outcomes. To effectively explore the dynamics of communication in the ICU, a study adopted a robust mixed-methods approach that allowed for a comprehensive understanding of clinicians' perceptions and experiences (see Ng et al., 2017). The surveys provided data on communication openness and related factors, offering a structured overview of trends and differences among the participants. Complementing this, the qualitative interviews delved deeper into the nuances of communication practices, revealing the contextual challenges and strategies employed by clinicians. Together, these methods enabled a holistic analysis, bridging statistical insights with first-hand narratives to uncover critical aspects of the ICU's communication culture.

This study, conducted in a public Hong Kong hospital ICU from October 2015 to September 2016, combined quantitative surveys with qualitative interviews. The ICU, a 21-bed closed unit, involved 80 participating clinicians, including doctors and nurses responsible for direct patient care. Ethical approval was secured, and participation was voluntary. The survey, adapted from Reader et al. (2007), assessed communication openness and related factors, such as leadership, satisfaction, and timeliness, using a validated and reliable instrument. Responses were analysed quantitatively using SPSS, and inferential statistics identified group differences in perceptions. Semi-structured interviews provided deeper insights into communication practices and challenges. In the surveyed ICU, teamwork quality and communication dynamics were evaluated through a validated survey involving 80 ICU staff members. The results highlighted differences in communication openness between doctors and nurses, shedding light on the underlying factors influencing these perceptions.

Key Findings About ICU Speak-Up Culture

The findings on communication openness reveal distinct dynamics between doctors and nurses in the ICU. Doctors reported greater comfort in speaking up, particularly within their teams during intradisciplinary interactions. They displayed confidence in raising concerns or seeking clarification among peers and superiors, which can be attributed to their perceived alignment of roles and shared professional identity. Furthermore, the hierarchical structure within the medical team seemed to pose fewer barriers for doctors, possibly due to the norms of medical practice that encourage question-driven discussions for decision-making. Conversely, nurses expressed lower levels of comfort in speaking up, especially in interdisciplinary settings involving doctors and other healthcare professionals. They often felt inhibited by hierarchical dynamics, which created significant barriers to open communication. Additionally, nurses highlighted specific challenges in voicing concerns during collaborative decision-making processes, where their input was perceived to carry less weight.

Several factors contributed to these dynamics. Hierarchical structures played a significant role, with power imbalances between doctors and nurses leading to the undervaluation of nurses' contributions, particularly during interdisciplinary discussions. Cultural norms, especially in settings influenced by traditional values, further exacerbated this issue, as respect for authority and seniority discouraged junior staff from challenging decisions or expressing dissenting opinions. Training and support disparities were also evident; while doctors had greater access to communication and leadership training, nurses often lacked training in assertive communication, which contributed to their hesitance in speaking up. Team dynamics further influenced communication openness, with stronger peer-to-peer relationships facilitating open dialogue, whereas poor team cohesion increased reluctance to engage.

To address these challenges, the findings suggest targeted interventions to bridge the communication gap between doctors and nurses. Fostering a non-blaming culture is essential to creating an environment where all team members feel valued and respected. Providing role-specific training tailored to nurses can equip them with the skills and confidence needed for high-stakes discussions. Reducing hierarchical barriers through policies that promote equality in interdisciplinary communication and decision-making processes is crucial. Strengthening team relationships through activities that build trust and mutual understanding among clinicians can also enhance communication openness. By addressing these issues, the ICU can cultivate a robust speak-up culture, improve teamwork, reduce errors, and ultimately elevate patient care outcomes.

Factors That Affect Speak-Up Culture in an ICU

The integration of audio-recorded observations and semi-structured interviews provided a richer, more nuanced understanding of the factors shaping communication practices within the ICU. These methods allowed the researchers to move beyond quantitative data, offering direct insights into the lived experiences of clinicians. By focusing on individuals identified as highly open communicators, the study uncovered key barriers, critical moments, and motivations influencing the speak-up culture. The findings revealed the interplay of hierarchical structures, time constraints, and cultural norms that shape communication dynamics, while also highlighting the pivotal role of patient safety, effective handovers, and leadership support in fostering an environment where clinicians feel empowered to voice concerns. This deeper exploration connects individual behaviours to broader systemic factors, underscoring the complexity of promoting effective communication in high-risk clinical settings. To gain deeper insights, ten individuals identified as having high communication openness were invited to participate in audio-recorded observations of their clinical practices.

Several factors were identified as impacting the speak-up culture in the ICU. First, hierarchical structures were a significant barrier, with both doctors and nurses acknowledging that these power dynamics often impeded open communication, especially during interdisciplinary interactions. Workload and time pressure also played a critical role, as the demands of high patient loads and tight schedules left little room for comprehensive discussions and collaborative decision-making. Additionally, cultural norms emphasizing respect for seniority discouraged junior staff from raising concerns, further complicating efforts to establish an environment of open communication.

Second, critical moments for speaking up in the ICU were identified, with patient safety concerns being the most prominent trigger for clinicians to voice issues. When potential risks to patient safety were identified, speaking up became essential to mitigate harm. Clinical handovers were another critical juncture, as the exchange of information during these transitions was pivotal for ensuring clarity and accuracy in communication. Additionally, interdisciplinary consultations between ICU staff and external departments often required assertiveness and clarification to address complex patient needs and ensure seamless collaboration.

Third, motivations for effective speak-up practices were closely linked to several key factors. Strong team dynamics played a vital role, with clinicians reporting greater confidence in speaking up when they had positive relationships within their teams. Training and experience also contributed significantly; clinicians who had undergone communication training or had extensive clinical experience felt better prepared to engage in open dialogue. Furthermore, supportive leadership was a critical motivator, as leaders who encouraged open communication and valued input from all staff levels created an environment conducive to fostering a robust speak-up culture.

Building on the key factors that motivate effective speak-up practices, it is essential to translate these insights into actionable strategies to enhance communication in critical care settings. The interplay between strong team dynamics, effective training, and supportive leadership underscores the need for a holistic approach to fostering a secure communication environment. By strengthening these foundational elements, healthcare teams can foster an environment where open dialogue and mutual respect flourish, paving the way for enhanced patient safety and improved care outcomes. The next section provides practical recommendations for achieving this goal within the ICU, with a focus on strategies designed to encourage communication openness and strengthen teamwork.

Comparative Perspectives on Speak-Up Cultures

Examining speak-up cultures across different countries or regions reveals how variations in organizational structures, cultural values, and healthcare policies influence communication dynamics in ICUs. For instance, Western healthcare systems often emphasize individual autonomy and open communication, which align with a lower tolerance for hierarchical barriers. This cultural alignment supports junior staff in voicing safety concerns without fear of reprisal. Conversely, in Asian contexts, including Hong Kong, respect for authority and seniority is deeply ingrained, creating additional challenges for fostering open dialogue. Comparative studies demonstrate that initiatives to promote a speak-up culture must account for these contextual differences. For example, while structured training programmes have proven effective in Western settings, they may need to be adapted in Asia to incorporate culturally sensitive approaches that bridge traditional values with modern teamwork practices.

Integrating global perspectives allows for the identification of best practices and innovative solutions that transcend cultural boundaries. For example, Scandinavian healthcare models focus on flat hierarchies and shared decision-making, which contribute to greater trust and transparency among team members. Such practices could serve as benchmarks for adapting communication strategies in Hong Kong's ICUs. Additionally, understanding how peer support systems are used in regions with high psychological safety could inspire similar interventions tailored to the Hong Kong context. By analysing these comparative frameworks, the chapter can highlight strategies that not only address local challenges but also leverage global insights to enhance ICU communication practices.

The Role of Technology in ICU Communication

Technological advancements offer opportunities to strengthen communication within ICUs, addressing challenges such as time constraints, documentation accuracy, and interdisciplinary collaboration. Tools like electronic health records (EHRs) and team communication platforms (e.g., secure messaging apps) can streamline information sharing and ensure that critical updates reach all relevant parties promptly. For example, a centralized digital system could facilitate real-time communication between doctors and nurses during patient handovers, minimizing errors caused by verbal omissions. Similarly, AI-driven diagnostic systems can support decision-making by providing evidence-based recommendations, enabling junior staff to voice concerns with data-driven confidence, which could mitigate hierarchical pressures.

However, the adoption of technology is not without its challenges. Over-reliance on digital tools can sometimes lead to depersonalized interactions, weakening the trust and rapport essential for a robust speak-up culture. Moreover, disparities in digital literacy among staff may exacerbate existing communication gaps, particularly for senior clinicians less familiar with new technologies. Therefore, implementing these tools must be accompanied by comprehensive training that ensures equitable access and integration into everyday workflows. By critically assessing the role of technology, this section underscores the dual potential of digital innovations to empower clinicians and foster an inclusive communication environment while addressing their limitations to avoid unintended consequences.

Psychological Safety and Burnout in Speak-Up Culture

Psychological safety, defined as the belief that one can voice concerns or make mistakes without fear of negative repercussions, plays a pivotal role in the speak-up culture of ICUs. When clinicians feel safe to express their thoughts, the likelihood of addressing safety concerns and improving teamwork increases significantly. This environment not only reduces the fear of retaliation but also promotes mutual respect among team members, which is particularly critical in high-stress settings like ICUs. By alleviating the pressure of conforming to hierarchical norms, psychological safety allows junior staff to engage more actively in decision-making processes, thus contributing to patient safety and staff satisfaction.

The link between psychological safety and burnout is particularly noteworthy in ICUs, where staff are exposed to high patient acuity, time pressures, and emotionally taxing situations. Burnout, characterized by emotional exhaustion and reduced professional efficacy, can severely undermine clinicians' ability to communicate effectively and speak up about safety issues. Addressing these concerns through initiatives such as resilience training, supportive leadership, and team-building activities can enhance psychological safety and mitigate burnout. Furthermore, fostering an open culture where staff feel valued and heard may lead to improved retention and overall well-being, ensuring a sustainable and effective workforce in critical care environments. By prioritizing psychological safety, ICUs can strengthen both staff resilience and the broader communication culture, ultimately enhancing patient care outcomes.

To build a truly effective communication culture in ICUs, it is essential to translate insights into actionable strategies that address both systemic and interpersonal dynamics. The preceding discussions on comparative perspectives, technological innovations, and psychological safety highlight the diverse factors that influence communication openness and the speak-up culture. Together, these elements emphasize the importance of integrating global best practices, leveraging digital tools thoughtfully, and fostering environments of trust and well-being. By addressing these interconnected aspects, healthcare teams can lay a robust foundation for improved teamwork and patient outcomes.

The next section consolidates these insights into specific, practical recommendations aimed at cultivating a secure and inclusive communication environment within the ICU. These strategies are designed to enhance openness, empower all team members, and establish a culture where collaboration and mutual respect thrive.

Recommendations for Fostering a Secure Communication Environment

To foster a secure communication environment in the ICU, a multifaceted approach is essential, encompassing strategies to enhance communication openness and teamwork. First, promoting equal status within teams is vital. This involves cultivating a non-hierarchical work culture where all members, regardless of their rank or role, feel valued and respected. For instance, junior nurses could be encouraged to share their observations during team meetings without fear of dismissal, reinforcing the idea that every perspective contributes to patient safety and care.

Second, providing regular communication training empowers clinicians to navigate complex interactions effectively. Such training should focus on assertiveness, conflict resolution, and culturally sensitive communication. For example, a workshop could include role-playing scenarios where participants practice addressing disagreements constructively, equipping them with skills to handle real-world challenges.

Third, leadership engagement is crucial for fostering open communication. Leaders should actively model transparent practices and create safe spaces where dialogue is welcomed. An example of this could be a senior doctor starting every shift with a team huddle, openly discussing potential challenges and encouraging team members to voice concerns or suggestions.

Fourth, implementing structured communication protocols such as ISBAR (Introduction, Situation, Background, Assessment, Recommendation) can standardize information exchange and reduce errors. For instance, during clinical handovers, using ISBAR ensures that critical patient information is consistently communicated, minimizing the risk of omissions.

Finally, addressing cultural barriers involves educating staff on how traditional norms may influence communication and encouraging a balance between cultural values and modern teamwork practices. For example, a training session could explore the impact of respect for hierarchy on communication openness, followed by group discussions on strategies to bridge generational and cultural gaps in a way that respects all parties. By integrating these strategies, hospital management and clinicians can work together to establish a more inclusive, effective, and secure communication environment in the ICU.

Conclusion

This chapter has explored the crucial role of speak-up culture in the Intensive Care Unit (ICU) of a Hong Kong hospital, focusing on the interplay between interdisciplinary (doctor-nurse) and intra-disciplinary (peer-to-peer) communication. Using a mixed-methods approach that includes cross-sectional surveys, audio-recorded observations, and semi-structured interviews, the study has identified key barriers and facilitators influencing communication openness, teamwork, and patient safety.

The findings reveal stark differences in how doctors and nurses perceive and engage in speaking up within the ICU. Doctors generally report greater confidence in voicing concerns, particularly within their own peer groups, reflecting a culture where decision-making and knowledge-sharing among medical professionals are normalized. However, this openness does not always extend to interdisciplinary interactions, where hierarchical structures and power imbalances can create tensions in communication.

For nurses, speaking up remains a significant challenge, especially in interactions with doctors. The study highlights three major barriers that contribute to communication reluctance. First, hierarchical workplace culture in Hong Kong and other Chinese settings emphasizes deference to seniority and professional status, leading many nurses to feel that their concerns are undervalued or dismissed. Second, cultural norms, particularly those influenced by Confucian values, discourage direct confrontation or dissent, even when patient safety is at risk. Unlike Western healthcare systems, where speaking up is encouraged as part of patient safety measures, the expectation in Hong Kong remains one of respect for authority and group harmony. Third, time constraints and clinical pressures in the fast-paced ICU environment leave little room for discussion, causing nurses to prioritize immediate task completion over questioning decisions. This leads to missed opportunities for collaborative problem-solving and knowledge exchange.

Despite these barriers, the chapter emphasizes that fostering a robust speak-up culture is essential for improving patient safety, enhancing interdisciplinary collaboration, and reducing medical errors in high-risk clinical environments. The findings align with broader research indicating that open communication in healthcare leads to higher staff satisfaction, reduced burnout, and better patient outcomes.

The challenges identified in this study are not unique to Hong Kong but are reflective of wider issues in ICUs globally, particularly in hierarchical medical cultures. A comparative analysis with Western and other Asian healthcare systems provides insights into how different institutional and cultural frameworks shape clinician communication practices. In Western healthcare systems such as the United States, the UK, and Scandinavia, emphasis is placed on flattened hierarchies and structured communication training to encourage junior staff to speak up. Regular training in assertive communication and patient safety protocols ensures that all team members feel empowered to raise concerns. In contrast, other Asian contexts, including Japan, South Korea, and Mainland China, face similar challenges where hierarchical workplace cultures prevent open dialogue. However, targeted interventions such as mandatory communication training, mentorship programmes, and leadership-driven cultural shifts have demonstrated some success in improving interdisciplinary communication.

By situating the findings within this global context, the chapter highlights potential models for addressing the identified barriers in Hong Kong's ICUs. Learning from best practices in Scandinavian and Australian ICUs, where teamwork and shared decision-making are prioritized, could offer valuable insights for developing localized interventions that balance cultural considerations with the need for improved communication.

One of the most critical factors influencing speak-up culture is leadership engagement. The study underscores the need for hospital administrators and senior clinicians to actively promote open communication, ensuring that all staff—regardless of rank—feel valued and heard. Leadership training and role modelling can help foster a non-punitive environment where feedback is welcomed, and errors are viewed as learning opportunities rather than grounds for punishment. Implementing structured communication frameworks such as SBAR (Situation, Background, Assessment, Recommendation) and closed-loop communication can also help standardize and normalize speaking up, reducing misunderstandings and power dynamics. Psychological safety initiatives that create an environment of mutual respect and trust are equally important, allowing team members to challenge unsafe practices, share concerns, and suggest alternative solutions.

While this study provides valuable insights into the barriers to speaking up in Hong Kong's ICU settings, further research is needed to explore the long-term impact of communication training and leadership interventions on speak-up culture and patient safety. Future research should also examine the role of mentorship and peer-support programmes in encouraging nurses and junior doctors to voice concerns. Additionally, the potential for technological innovations, such as real-time communication apps and AI-driven decision-support systems, to facilitate more transparent and efficient interdisciplinary communication should be explored.

Policy recommendations should be developed in collaboration with hospital management to ensure that communication improvements are institutionalized rather than dependent on individual effort. By addressing structural, cultural, and procedural barriers, healthcare institutions can create a sustainable framework for enhancing teamwork and patient safety in ICUs.

This chapter reinforces the critical role of speak-up culture in improving communication, collaboration, and patient safety in ICUs. By understanding the systemic, cultural, and professional challenges that hinder open communication, hospital administrators and clinicians can implement evidence-based strategies to bridge the communication gap. The recommendations put forth—leadership-driven initiatives, structured communication training, and fostering psychological safety—serve as actionable steps toward building a more inclusive and effective communication environment in high-stakes clinical settings. Beyond Hong Kong, the study's insights contribute to the broader discourse on communication in critical care, offering valuable lessons for ICUs worldwide. By integrating global best practices while tailoring interventions to local cultural contexts, healthcare institutions can create safer, more collaborative environments where speaking up is not just encouraged but embedded in everyday clinical practice.

References

Ayoko, O. B. (2007). Communication openness, conflict events and reactions to conflict in culturally diverse workgroups. *Cross Cultural Management: An International Journal, 14*, 105–124. https://doi.org/10.1108/13527600710745723

Law, B. Y., & Chan, E. A. (2015). The experience of learning to speak up: A narrative inquiry on newly graduated registered nurses. *Journal of Clinical Nursing, 24*, 1837–1848. https://doi.org/10.1111/jocn.12805

Leonard, M., Graham, S., & Bonacum, D. (2004). The human factor: The critical importance of effective teamwork and communication in providing safe care. *Quality & Safety in Health Care, 13*(1), i85–i90. https://doi.org/10.1136/qshc.2004.010033

Morrison, E. W., & Milliken, F. J. (2003). Speaking up, remaining silent: The dynamics of voice and silence in organizations. *Journal of Management Studies, 40*, 1353–1358. https://doi.org/10.1111/1467-6486.00383

Nembhard, I. M., Labao, I., & Savage, S. (2015). Breaking the silence: Determinants of voice for quality improvement in hospitals. *Health Care Management Review, 40*, 225–236. https://doi.org/10.1097/HMR.0000000000000028

Ng, G. W. Y., Pun, J., So, E. H. K., Chiu, W. W. H., Leung, A. S. H., Stone, Y. H., Lam, C. L., Lai, S. P. W., Leung, R. P. W., Luk, H. W., Leung, A. K. H., Au-Yeung, K. W., Lai, K. Y., Slade, D., & Chan, E. A. (2017). Exploring speaking-up culture in an intensive care unit (ICU): Chinese doctors' and nurses' perceptions of the openness of communication. *BMJ Open, 7*(8), e015721. https://doi.org/10.1136/bmjopen-2016-015721

Reader, T. W., Flin, R., Mearns, K., & Cuthbertson, B. H. (2007). Interdisciplinary communication in the intensive care unit. *British Journal of Anaesthesia, 98*, 347–352. https://doi.org/10.1093/bja/ael372

Rogers, P. C., Graham, C. R., & Mayes, C. T. (2007). Cultural competence and instructional design: Exploration research into the delivery of online instruction cross-culturally. *Educational Technology Research and Development, 55*, 197–217. https://doi.org/10.1007/s11423-007-9033-x

7

Teaching Clinical Communication to Medical Students in Hong Kong

Clinical Communication in Hong Kong Context

Clinical communication is at the heart of healthcare delivery, playing a critical role in the success of patient interactions, especially when sensitive topics such as delivering bad news or managing complex patient scenarios are involved (Fallowfield & Jenkins, 2004; Slade et al., 2008). Effective communication ensures that medical information is conveyed clearly, emotional needs are acknowledged, and patients feel supported throughout their healthcare journey (Back & Arnold, 2009; Nelson et al., 2005). For an example, in the Chinese context, doctors often prioritize involving family members in discussions about diagnosis and treatment plans, ensuring that medical information is conveyed not only to the patient but also to their family, while using culturally appropriate language to address emotional needs and provide reassurance (Pun et al., 2018). For instance, in the Hong Kong context, a doctor might address a patient's fear about a serious diagnosis by using the phrase "*唔使擔心*" ("don't worry") in Cantonese, followed by an explanation in simple, non-technical terms, while acknowledging the importance of family support by saying, "*我哋會同你嘅家人一齊商量下一步點做*" ("We will

J. Pun, *Exploring and Teaching Healthcare Communication*,
https://doi.org/10.1007/978-3-031-08675-5_7

discuss the next steps together with your family"), blending both emotional reassurance and cultural sensitivity to ensure the patient feels comforted and supported (See more Pun, 2023).

In Hong Kong, the healthcare landscape is shaped consistently by both Western medical practices and traditional Chinese culture, making the teaching of clinical communication uniquely challenging (Pun et al., 2018). This dual influence perhaps requires medical professionals, especially those novice medical students to navigate not only medical knowledge but also cultural expectations such as collective decision-making, the role of family in healthcare choices, and the preference for indirect communication when discussing sensitive topics like terminal illness, adding layers of complexity to teaching effective clinical communication in this context (Jha et al., 2015; Pun et al., 2021).

While medical students are typically trained in Western medical education following with Western style of communication protocols or guidelines, these approaches often fail to account for the local cultural and linguistic nuances of Hong Kong (Pun et al., 2018). For instance, Chinese patients frequently expect family involvement in medical decision-making, which contrasts with the individual-cantered approach of Western medicine. For an example, a Chinese patient was diagnosed with a serious illness. He involved his entire family in deciding on surgery, emphasizing the collective family perspective, which contrasts with the Western approach of expecting individual decision-making. Additionally, communication around terminal illnesses or End-of-Life (EOL) in Chinese culture tends to be more euphemistic and indirect, further complicating the application of Western frameworks (Pun et al., 2021). This chapter explores the complexities of teaching clinical communication to medical students in Hong Kong, examining the current models in use, the gaps in existing teaching approaches, and the potential for a more culturally responsive framework.

Teaching Clinical Communication Frameworks in Hong Kong Context

Clinical communication models, such as the SPIKES framework and the Calgary-Cambridge guide, have been widely adopted in medical schools across Hong Kong (Pun, 2023). The SPIKES (Setting, Perception, Invitation, Knowledge, Empathy, Summarize or Strategy) framework is designed to guide doctors in delivering bad news to patients through a structured six-step approach (i.e., Setting up, Perception, Invitation, Knowledge, Emotions, Strategy and Summary), from setting up the interview to handling the patient's emotional response, while the Calgary-Cambridge model offers a comprehensive guide for medical consultations, emphasizing patient-centred communication and building rapport throughout the clinical interaction (Mallinson, 2023). These models, developed in English-speaking world, emphasize perhaps key components such as empathy, structured delivery of information, and patient engagement during critical conversations. Still, many studies from East Asia suggest that these models may be tailored primarily for Western audiences, where direct communication and individual decision-making are the norm (Betsch et al., 2016; Pun et al., 2018). For instance, in Western contexts, when a patient receives a cancer diagnosis, the doctor typically provides all the information directly, and the patient is expected to make treatment decisions independently, involving family members only if they choose to. In contrast, within the Chinese context, where patients often depend significantly on family members for emotional, financial support and decision-making when receiving difficult news, these frameworks perhaps may not fully address their communication needs in Chinese context. Such cultural expectations surrounding end-of-life discussions also differ significantly. For instance, Chinese families often prefer to shield patients from harsh realities, such as terminal diagnoses, prognosis, or estimated life expectancy, which contrasts with the Western emphasis on full disclosure and patient autonomy (Pun, 2021a, 2021b, 2021c).

A growing number of studies have indirectly suggested that Hong Kong medical students, regardless of their clinical disciplines or training, although well-versed in these Western communication protocols, struggle to apply them effectively in local clinical settings (Pun, 2022). One key challenge is the language barrier. Many students are more comfortable delivering clinical information in English, but building rapport and expressing empathy in Cantonese—a local language with its own set of cultural values and expressions—is where the difficulty lies. In Hong Kong's clinical environments, bilingual hospital staff—primarily native Cantonese speakers trained in English—often lack familiarity with Chinese written medical terminology, leading to a practice where medical records are written in English, patient communication occurs in Cantonese, and staff frequently code-switch or engage in translanguaging between spoken Cantonese and medical English (Pun, 2021c). As a result, translanguaging, or the switching between English for medical terms and Cantonese for general conversation, perhaps can confuse patients and disrupt the flow of communication (Pun, 2021a, 2021b, 2021c).

One study has explored how hospital staff in Hong Kong manage clinical handovers in a bilingual context, using both Cantonese and English. Through interviews with 78 doctors and nurses, the study identified challenges in translanguaging—switching between languages during handovers—that can lead to information loss or ambiguity, especially when communicating with non-native speakers and elderly patients. Pun's study (2021a) underscores the importance of communication structured protocols like ISBAR to standardize communication and suggests that targeted training can enhance bilingual handover practices, reducing risks and improving patient safety (Pun, 2021a). The nuances of Cantonese and the expectations around non-verbal communication complicate these interactions (Pun, 2021a, 2021b, 2021c). The bilingual nature of hospital staff, who frequently switch between Cantonese and English for both patient interaction and professional communication, further complicates the teaching of clinical communication by requiring medical professionals to navigate not only linguistic challenges but also the nuanced interplay of language, medical terminology, and cultural expectations (Pun, 2021b). This complexity is further amplified by Hong Kong's sociocultural context, where deeply rooted cultural values and family dynamics significantly influence clinical communication and decision-making processes.

Hong Kong's Sociocultural Context

The sociocultural environment in Hong Kong presents a unique set of challenges for clinical communication. The influence of Confucian values, particularly filial piety, dictates that family members often play a central role in decision-making processes. The hierarchical nature of these family structures means that older family members, not necessarily the patients, are often involved in determining the course of treatment (Pun et al., 2018). Additionally, there is a cultural aversion to discussing death and terminal illness directly. Euphemistic language is frequently used to soften the emotional impact of bad news. Medical students, therefore, need to navigate these cultural expectations while balancing the ethical need for transparency and patient-centred care (Pun, 2022; Pun, Yu, & Lee, 2022). The role of the family and the preference for indirect communication complicates direct patient-doctor conversations, especially when students attempt to apply Western communication frameworks (Pun, 2021a, 2021b, 2021c). An example of indirect communication very common to be found in Hong Kong context is that when a family member, usually the carer, speaks on behalf of the patient, conveying the patient's needs or concerns without directly addressing sensitive topics such as the severity of an illness, to avoid distressing the patient. Instead of discussing the prognosis openly, they might use vague or softened language, or shift the focus to treatment options without explicitly acknowledging the full gravity of the situation. Consequently, the patient may not receive complete or accurate information about their condition, leading to misunderstandings, reduced patient autonomy, and potentially less effective decision-making regarding their own care and treatment options (Iconomou et al., 2002). For the clinician, this indirect communication can create difficulties in building trust, accurately assessing the patient's understanding of their condition, ultimately complicating the delivery of appropriate and effective care (Thorne et al., 2008).

Teaching Clinical Communication in Hong Kong

One of the most significant challenges that Hong Kong medical students face is the linguistic landscape divides between Cantonese and English. Although many medical students are proficient in English, often due to their education in international schools or English-medium public-funded secondary schools—the primary language of instruction in medical programmes—they are still expected to communicate with patients predominantly in Cantonese (Pun, 2023). Some of these students perhaps have minimal exposure to Cantonese, both in their academic environment and in their daily lives, resulting in limited opportunities to develop proficiency in the language. This presents a challenge because medical students may be adept at explaining medical terms in English but struggle with the cultural and emotional nuances of Cantonese (Pun et al., 2015). For example, while a medical student may be able to describe a diagnosis like "abdominal pain" in English, they might struggle to understand or interpret the specific type of abdominal pain being described by a patient in Cantonese, making it difficult to accurately diagnose or explain the condition using appropriate medical terminology. Students may also find it challenging to use the appropriate Cantonese terms or expressions that convey the condition in a culturally sensitive manner, particularly when communicating with elderly patients who might prefer familiar colloquial language or hold traditional health beliefs (Cordella et al., 2014). Students have reported difficulties in using Cantonese to express empathy and build rapport, even though they can competently convey clinical information (Pun, 2021a, 2021b, 2021c). This lack of fluency in emotionally sensitive communication impacts their ability to connect with patients on a personal level. The gap between these frameworks and local cultural practices creates challenges for medical students, who are often unsure of how to involve family members without undermining patient autonomy or how to balance the need for truth-telling with the local preference for indirect communication (Pun, 2022). To explore these challenges further and understand how medical students navigate them in practice, the next section will elaborate a study conducted by Pun (2021b) which explores how Chinese medical students in Hong Kong deliver bad news and their communication patterns.

Case Study: Scenario-Based Role-Play in Delivering Bad News

In medical education, the ability to communicate effectively and compassionately, especially when delivering bad news, is a critical skill for future doctors (Rosenbaum et al., 2004). The complexities of these conversations are magnified in multicultural contexts, like Hong Kong, where language, cultural norms, and expectations influence how medical information is conveyed and received. This case study by Pun (2021c) examines how final-year medical students at a medical school in Hong Kong manage the delicate task of delivering bad news within a simulated clinical environment, shedding light on the challenges they face and the strategies they employ.

Context

At the heart of this study is the "Serious Illness Communication Module," an integral part of the curriculum for Year-6 medical students at one of the medical schools in Hong Kong. A total of 50 students voluntarily participated, immersing themselves in scenario-based role-play exercises designed to simulate the delivery of critical medical diagnoses. Each exercise required students to engage in 20-minute critical conversations, conducted entirely in Cantonese, the local language. The goal was to mirror real-world situations as closely as possible, allowing students to practice delivering emotionally charged news while managing the linguistic and cultural nuances specific to the Hong Kong healthcare setting.

The study adopted a qualitative, cross-sectional observational design, adhering to the Strengthening the Reporting of Observational Studies in Epidemiology (STROBE) protocol to ensure rigor and reliability. The role-play sessions were meticulously planned, featuring professional actors who portrayed patients and their family members. These actors were trained to create realistic scenarios, imitating common interactions encountered in clinical practice. The inclusion of family members in these scenarios is particularly relevant, as decision-making in the Hong Kong context often involves multiple family stakeholders. This setup provided students with an immersive and authentic learning experience, enabling them to engage with the complexities of culturally sensitive communication.

Data Collection

To capture the intricacies of these interactions, the role-play sessions were video-recorded, supplemented with detailed field notes that documented non-verbal cues such as body language, tone, and gestures—critical components of effective communication. Each session, lasting approximately 10 minutes, involved multiple participants: a student doctor, an actor playing a patient's family member, and a senior consultant (also portrayed by an actor). The recordings were subsequently transcribed and translated into English to facilitate comprehensive analysis. To ensure the accuracy and reliability of the data, two clinicians—a critical care physician and a geriatrician—verified the transcripts. These clinicians also served as educators within the course, adding another layer of expertise. Additionally, a research assistant cross-checked the transcripts against the video recordings to maintain consistency and precision.

Analysis

An ethnographic discourse analysis was employed to deconstruct the sequences of interaction between the students and simulated patients. This method allowed for a deep dive into the nuances of communication, focusing on how students initiated conversations, responded to patients' and family members' emotions, and adapted their communication strategies based on the patients' and families' cues. Special attention was paid to the students' use of language, examining elements such as turn-taking, pauses, and question types, which are essential in understanding how effectively empathy and information were communicated.

The analysis was conducted in two stages. Initially, a coding framework was developed through discussions with healthcare professionals, who provided insights into effective communication practices in clinical settings. This framework guided the subsequent coding process, which involved two independent raters who reviewed 10% of the data to ensure the reliability of the coding scheme. This dual-stage process aimed to capture the diversity of communication styles and to identify recurring patterns in how students approached the delivery of bad news.

Findings: Identifying Medical Students' Communication Patterns in Hong Kong

The analysis revealed six key discourse strategies that students employed during their interactions:

1. **Emphasizing Patients' Emotional Needs**: Some students showed an awareness of the emotional impact of the news and prioritized addressing patients' feelings before discussing medical details.
2. **Balancing Medical and Emotional Information**: Others attempted to present information in a way that balanced the technical aspects of the diagnosis with empathetic responses to patients' emotional states.
3. **Directing Attention to Treatment Options**: Some students directed the conversation towards actionable next steps, helping patients focus on future plans rather than solely on the bad news.
4. **Acknowledging Patients' Physical Discomfort and Wishes**: This strategy involved recognizing the physical and psychological impact of the diagnosis and aligning the treatment discussion with patients' preferences and comfort levels.
5. **Directly Disclosing Bad News**: A few students adhered strictly to Western models, such as the SPIKES protocol, delivering the news directly, but often struggling to soften the impact or provide adequate emotional support.

6. **Addressing Family Expectations**: Given the cultural context, some students attempted to engage with the family members present, reflecting the collective decision-making practices typical in Hong Kong's healthcare system.

These strategies underscored an awareness among the students of the need to cater not only to the patients' informational needs but also to their emotional and familial concerns. However, the effectiveness of these strategies varied, highlighting areas for improvement in medical training.

Challenges of Adapting Western Communication Models in Hong Kong Context

The findings highlighted a significant challenge faced by the students: the adaptation of Western-based communication models to the local Hong Kong context. While many students attempted to follow established protocols such as the SPIKES model, these frameworks were not always compatible with the cultural expectations prevalent in Hong Kong. The emphasis on direct communication in Western models often clashed with the preference for indirectness in Chinese society, especially when discussing sensitive issues like terminal illnesses. The students' attempts to convey empathy frequently appeared mechanical, lacking the genuine, culturally appropriate expressions of care crucial for effective communication in the local context. For example, when explaining a diagnosis, many students used English medical terminology, as they had been trained in English-speaking environments. However, they often reverted to Cantonese for brief social exchanges, leading to disruptions in the communication flow. This inconsistency not only confused patients but also undermined the students' efforts to build rapport and trust.

Another major challenge was the engagement of family members, a crucial aspect of healthcare interactions in Hong Kong. The Western frameworks students followed primarily focused on direct patient-doctor communication, leaving them underprepared for scenarios where family involvement was necessary. In Chinese society, families play a central role in decision-making, particularly in end-of-life care, where family members often decide what information to disclose to the patient. Students struggled with using indirect language and euphemisms, culturally appropriate methods for discussing terminal illnesses, illustrating the gap between their training and the realities of clinical practice in Hong Kong (Pun, 2023). The results of this study emphasize the need for culturally responsive training frameworks that incorporate local communication practices. To better prepare medical students for the realities of clinical practice in Hong Kong, medical schools must move beyond Western models and integrate culturally specific communication strategies. This approach includes training students in the use of indirect language, appropriate use of Cantonese medical terminology, and techniques for effectively engaging family members in critical conversations. Enhancing role-play exercises with these elements can help bridge the gap between theoretical knowledge and practical application, ensuring that future doctors are equipped to deliver bad news in a way that is both effective and culturally sensitive.

Proposed Framework for Clinical Communication Training in Hong Kong: Culturally Appropriate Protocols

The findings from the case study reveal a significant gap between the Western-based communication models currently taught and the real-world needs of medical students in Hong Kong. While frameworks such as the SPIKES and Calgary-Cambridge guides provide a structured method for delivering bad news, they often fall short in addressing the cultural and linguistic complexities inherent in Hong Kong's healthcare system. The study highlighted how final-year medical students, despite their familiarity with these Western models, struggled to adapt their approaches effectively, underscoring the need for a culturally responsive and hybrid framework that integrates local practices. In Hong Kong, healthcare conversations are deeply influenced by cultural values such as collective decision-making, filial piety, and indirect communication.

Patients and their families expect medical professionals to approach sensitive topics like terminal illnesses with a high degree of tact and respect, often involving the entire family in the decision-making process. This expectation contrasts sharply with the more individual-focused, direct communication emphasized in Western frameworks. Therefore, to bridge this gap, the integration of culturally specific communication strategies—such as understanding family hierarchies, using indirect language, and employing euphemisms when discussing end-of-life care—could enhance the relevance and applicability of these frameworks in Hong Kong's context (see more from Pun et al., 2021).

For instance, rather than conveying a terminal diagnosis explicitly, healthcare professionals might discuss "treatment options" without directly addressing the prognosis, thus aligning with local preferences for indirect communication. This approach is not about withholding information but rather about presenting it in a manner that respects the patient's and family's cultural expectations (Pun, 2021a, 2022). Such strategies are essential for creating a compassionate and supportive environment that builds trust between patients, families, and healthcare providers. The importance of understanding family dynamics in Hong Kong's context cannot be understated. The cultural principle of filial piety and collective decision-making means that family members often play a central role in treatment decisions. Training medical students to engage with both the patient and their families is critical. This involves teaching them how to diplomatically negotiate with family members and incorporate their input without compromising the patient's autonomy. Integrating these skills into the curriculum will better prepare students for the realities of clinical scenarios in Hong Kong, where the family's role is not only expected but vital.

Enhancing Communication Skills: Medical Cantonese and Translanguaging Practices

To develop these competencies, targeted training should focus on medical Cantonese, as the study demonstrated that students frequently struggled with translating technical information and expressing empathy in the local language. Cantonese, with its rich set of cultural expressions and nuances, is crucial for building rapport and engaging patients effectively. Training students to navigate these subtleties is essential; they must not only translate medical terminology into accessible Cantonese but also choose the appropriate expressions that convey empathy and support. For example, understanding when and how to use phrases like "唔使擔心" ("don't worry") in a culturally sensitive manner can significantly impact patient outcomes and satisfaction (Pun, 2021a). Moreover, as much of the technical training is conducted in English, students need to become proficient in translanguaging (Pun, 2021c)—seamlessly transitioning between English and Cantonese during consultations. This bilingual approach ensures that communication remains clear, compassionate, and culturally competent. Training students to navigate these linguistic transitions effectively can help them build trusting relationships with patients and families, ensuring that medical information is conveyed accurately while maintaining a supportive atmosphere.

Role-Play and Reflective Learning

Scenario-based role-play exercises have proven to be a fundamental component of clinical communication training, offering students the opportunity to practice their skills in a controlled and realistic environment (Lavanya et al., 2024). The study's findings support the continuation and expansion of such exercises but emphasize the need for supplementary real-time feedback and reflective learning opportunities to enhance their effectiveness (Bardach et al., 2021). Incorporating video analysis of student-patient interactions can be particularly powerful. Recording role-play sessions allows students to review their verbal and non-verbal communication patterns, enabling them to identify areas for improvement, such as body language, tone of voice, and choice of language (Bagacean et al., 2020). Peer and instructor feedback can provide a comprehensive perspective, helping students refine their techniques and increase their cultural sensitivity (Wang & Li, 2011). For instance, peers might offer insights into how effectively a student managed to maintain eye contact or showed empathy during a difficult conversation, while instructors can provide expert advice on aligning language use with cultural and family expectations.

Reflective practice sessions following role-plays encourage students to critically analyse their performance (Kilgour et al., 2015). This reflection not only allows students to consider what went well but also to think through what they could do differently in future interactions. For example, after reviewing a role-play scenario, a student might reflect on how they could have used more culturally appropriate language when explaining a diagnosis or engaged the family members more actively in the discussion. This iterative process of practice, feedback, and reflection fosters deeper learning and helps students internalize communication strategies that are both effective and culturally sensitive (Hutchins & Goldstein Hode, 2021). Recognizing the central role that families play in healthcare decision-making in Hong Kong is also vital. Medical students need to learn how to engage families respectfully while safeguarding patient autonomy (Pun et al., 2021). Practical exercises that simulate scenarios involving family-inclusive decision-making will help students develop these essential skills. For instance, role-play exercises could include situations where a family member takes the lead in the conversation, requiring the student to navigate this dynamic while ensuring that the patient's voice is still heard and respected. Additionally, training should include scenarios that reflect the complexity of negotiating with families who may prefer not to disclose the full extent of an illness to the patient. These simulations help students practice balancing cultural expectations with ethical considerations, such as informed consent and patient autonomy, preparing them to manage these challenging conversations with professionalism and sensitivity (Cavallaro & Sridhar, 2020).

Conclusion: Integrating Cultural Competence into Medical Education

The chapter details the integration of culturally informed communication training within Hong Kong's medical education system, emphasizing the need for culturally responsive practices beyond traditional Western models. It highlights the challenges faced by medical students in adapting frameworks like SPIKES and the Calgary-Cambridge guide to Hong Kong's sociocultural context, where indirect communication, family involvement, and linguistic diversity are crucial. The chapter proposes a hybrid communication framework that combines Western models with local adaptations, focusing on improving students' abilities in translanguaging, role-play, and scenario-based reflective learning to enhance patient-centred care.

The evidence from the role-play study strongly supports the need for a shift in Hong Kong's medical education programmes towards integrating culturally informed communication training methods. By addressing both the technical and cultural aspects of clinical communication, these programmes can better prepare students for the realities of practice, ensuring that they are not only equipped with technical knowledge but also the linguistic and cultural competencies necessary to provide effective, patient-centred care in a multicultural and bilingual environment. In summary, integrating culturally appropriate protocols, enhancing language skills through translanguaging practices, and incorporating reflective, scenario-based learning can transform clinical communication training. This approach ensures that medical students are prepared to engage with patients and families effectively, meeting the diverse and culturally nuanced needs of Hong Kong's healthcare system.

References

Back, A., & Arnold, R. (2009). *Mastering Communication with Seriously Ill Patients: Balancing Honesty with Empathy and Hope.* Cambridge University Press.

Bagacean, C., Cousin, I., Ubertini, A. H., El Yacoubi El Idrissi, M., Bordron, A., Mercadie, L., et al. (2020). Simulated patient and role play methodologies for communication skills and empathy training of undergraduate medical students. *BMC Medical Education, 20*, 1–8.

Bardach, L., Klassen, R. M., Durksen, T. L., Rushby, J. V., Bostwick, K. C., & Sheridan, L. (2021). The power of feedback and reflection: Testing an online scenario-based learning intervention for student teachers. *Computers & Education, 169*, 104194.

Betsch, C., Böhm, R., Airhihenbuwa, C. O., Butler, R., Chapman, G. B., Haase, N., et al. (2016). Improving medical decision making and health promotion through culture-sensitive health communication: An agenda for science and practice. *Medical Decision Making, 36*(7), 811–833.

Cavallaro, J. L., & Sridhar, M. (2020). Reducing bias in human rights fact-finding: The potential of the clinical simulation model to overcome ethical, practical, and cultural tensions in "foreign" contexts. *Human Rights Quarterly, 42*(2), 488–512.

Cordella, M., Poiani, A., Cordella, M., & Poiani, A. (2014). Language and the cross-cultural dimension of cancer. In *Behavioural Oncology: Psychological, Communicative, and Social Dimensions* (pp. 351–460).

Fallowfield, L., & Jenkins, V. (2004). Communicating sad, bad, and difficult news in medicine. *The Lancet, 363*(9405), 312–319.

Hutchins, D., & Goldstein Hode, M. (2021). Exploring faculty and staff development of cultural competence through communicative learning in an online diversity course. *Journal of Diversity in Higher Education, 14*(4), 468.

Iconomou, G., Viha, A., Koutras, A., Vagenakis, A. G., & Kalofonos, H. P. (2002). Information needs and awareness of diagnosis in patients with cancer receiving chemotherapy: A report from Greece. *Palliative Medicine, 16*(4), 315–321.

Jha, V., Mclean, M., Gibbs, T. J., & Sandars, J. (2015). Medical professionalism across cultures: A challenge for medicine and medical education. *Medical Teacher, 37*(1), 74–80.

Kilgour, P., Reynaud, D., Northcote, M. T., & Shields, M. (2015). Role-playing as a tool to facilitate learning, self-reflection and social awareness in teacher education. *International Journal of Innovative Interdisciplinary Research, 2*(4), 8–20.

Lavanya, K. M., Somu, L. K., & Mishra, S. K. (2024). Effectiveness of scenario-based roleplay as a method of teaching soft skills for undergraduate medical students. *International Journal of Applied and Basic Medical Research, 14*(2), 78–84.

Mallinson, T. (2023). Consultation skills and the diagnostic process. In *Primary Care for Paramedics.*

Nelson, J. E., Kinjo, K., Meier, D. E., Ahmad, K., & Morrison, R. S. (2005). When critical illness becomes chronic: Informational needs of patients and families. *Journal of Critical Care, 20*(1), 79–89.

Pun, J. (2021a). Clinical handover in a bilingual setting: Interpretative phenomenological analysis to exploring translanguaging practices for effective communication among hospital staff. *BMJ Open, 11*, e046494, 1–9.

Pun, J. (2021b). A study of Chinese medical students' communication pattern in delivering bad news: An ethnographic discourse analysis approach. *BMC Medical Education, 21*(286), 1–10.

Pun, J. (2021c). Factors associated with nurses' perceptions, their communication skills and the quality of clinical handover in the Hong Kong context. *BMC Nursing, 20*(95), 1–8.

Pun, J. (2022). The priorities, challenges, and scope of clinical communication teaching perceived by clinicians from different disciplines: A Hong Kong case study. *BMC Primary Care, 22*, 158, 1–16.

Pun, J. (2023). *The Role of Language in Eastern and Western Health Communication.* Routledge.

Pun, J., Matthiessen, C. M. I. M., Slade, D., & Murray, K. (2015). Factors affecting communication in emergency departments: Doctors and nurses' perceptions of communication in a trilingual ED in Hong Kong. *International Journal of Emergency Medicine, 8*, 48.

Pun, J. K., Chan, E. A., Wang, S., & Slade, D. (2018). Health professional-patient communication practices in East Asia: An integrative review of an emerging field of research and practice in Hong Kong, South Korea, Japan, Taiwan, and Mainland China. *Patient Education and Counseling, 101*(7), 1193–1206.

Pun, J., Cheung, K. M., & Chow, C. H. J. (2021). A systematic review of teaching end of life communication: The priorities, the challenges and the scope. *BMJ Supportive & Palliative Care, 12*(4), 368–375.

Pun, J., Yu, Q. J., & Lee, M. K. C. (2022). An ethnographic discourse approach to explore GP-counsellor communication in primary health care settings in Hong Kong. *Frontiers in Psychology, 13*, 943840. https://doi.org/10.3389/fpsyg.2022.943840

Rosenbaum, M. E., Ferguson, K. J., & Lobas, J. G. (2004). Teaching medical students and residents skills for delivering bad news: A review of strategies. *Academic Medicine, 79*(2), 107–117.

Slade, D., Scheeres, H., Manidis, M., Iedema, R., Dunston, R., Stein-Parbury, J., et al. (2008). Emergency communication: The discursive challenges facing emergency clinicians and patients in hospital emergency departments. *Discourse & Communication, 2*(3), 271–298.

Thorne, S. E., Hislop, T. G., Armstrong, E. A., & Oglov, V. (2008). Cancer care communication: The power to harm and the power to heal? *Patient Education and Counseling, 71*(1), 34–40.

Wang, T., & Li, L. Y. (2011). 'Tell me what to do' vs. 'guide me through it': Feedback experiences of international doctoral students. *Active Learning in Higher Education, 12*(2), 101–112.

8

Educating Medical Students in Hong Kong on Clinical Communication: Emphasizing End-of-Life Conversations

Navigating End-of-Life Communication in Hong Kong

Effective clinical communication is a cornerstone of quality healthcare, particularly in culturally diverse and complex environments such as Hong Kong. As medical students transition into professional practice, their ability to communicate clearly, empathetically, and effectively becomes increasingly vital. This is especially true when addressing sensitive subjects such as end-of-life (EOL) care, where conversations often encompass discussions about treatment options, prognosis, and patients' final wishes. In these situations, the way information is communicated can significantly influence patients' emotional well-being, treatment choices, and overall quality of care. Hong Kong presents a unique context for teaching EOL communication due to its multicultural healthcare environment, where Western medical practices coexist with traditional Chinese values and practices. As a result, clinicians must navigate a complex landscape that balances Western principles, such as patient autonomy and transparency, with Chinese cultural priorities, such as family involvement, filial piety, and the emphasis on maintaining harmony (Pun

J. Pun, *Exploring and Teaching Healthcare Communication*,
https://doi.org/10.1007/978-3-031-08675-5_8

et al., 2018, 2020). Chinese culture traditionally views death as a taboo topic, often leading to hesitancy among clinicians and families to engage in open conversations about EOL issues. This reluctance is compounded by cultural practices like "collusion," where families request that clinicians withhold distressing information from patients to protect them emotionally (Pun et al., 2023).

Despite the prevalence of Western communication frameworks, such as the SPIKES protocol (Setting, Perception, Invitation, Knowledge, Empathy, and Summary) and the Calgary-Cambridge guide, these models are perhaps insufficient in addressing the nuances of EOL discussions in Hong Kong (Pun, 2023). These models, designed primarily for Western contexts, emphasize patient autonomy and direct, transparent communication—approaches that may not align with the cultural and familial expectations in Hong Kong's predominantly Chinese society (Pun et al., 2018). For instance, in Chinese culture, the family often assumes a central role in decision-making, and patients may defer important healthcare decisions to their relatives, believing that this fulfils their cultural and moral obligations (Pun et al., 2020, 2023). This chapter highlights the need for a culturally adapted model of teaching clinical communication in Hong Kong, particularly for EOL care. It argues that existing Western models must be adapted and integrated with culturally specific practices to be effective in this unique context. A hybrid approach that combines Western techniques with Chinese communication practices can provide medical students with a more comprehensive understanding of how to navigate EOL conversations. This integrated approach respects the cultural norms of family involvement and patient deference while ensuring that the patient's rights and needs remain central (Pun et al., 2018, 2020). Furthermore, local studies and systematic reviews demonstrate that integrating both Western and Chinese models into medical education can significantly improve outcomes. By understanding the intricacies of EOL communication within Hong Kong's healthcare system, educators can better equip medical students to manage the complex dynamics of these conversations. This involves not only imparting the technical skills needed to communicate about treatment options and prognoses but also emphasizing the importance of cultural sensitivity and empathy (Pun et al., 2018, 2023).

Given these challenges and opportunities, this chapter aims to provide a comprehensive framework for teaching EOL communication that is tailored to Hong Kong's healthcare context. It explores the cultural factors influencing EOL discussions, the role of family in medical decision-making, and the limitations of applying Western models in isolation. Additionally, the chapter discusses practical teaching strategies—such as simulated patient encounters, role-playing with real-life cases, and interdisciplinary collaboration—that can prepare students for the multifaceted nature of EOL communication. By developing these skills, medical students will be better equipped to provide patient-centred, culturally sensitive care that enhances the quality of EOL care and supports the diverse needs of Hong Kong's patient population (Pun et al., 2021, 2023). This chapter explores the need for a culturally appropriate model of teaching clinical communication in Hong Kong, with a focus on EOL conversations. Drawing from systematic reviews and local studies, this chapter discusses the intricacies of EOL communication, the role of family in decision-making, and the importance of integrating both Western and Chinese communication models into medical education.

The Role of End-of-Life Communication

End-of-life (EOL) communication is perhaps very challenging for medical professionals especially those junior or without much experience to deal with life-and-death situation, involving crucial discussions about a patient's prognosis, and their plans for approaching the end of life. A common definition for end-of-life communication refers to the communication process of discussing a patient's health condition, treatment choices, and preferences for care as they near the end of their life (Anselm et al., 2005; Sinuff et al., 2015). It involves medical professionals, the patient, and their family, aiming to ensure that care decisions align with the patient's wishes and provide emotional support during this difficult time. To illustrate the complexities and sensitivities involved in EOL communication, the following case study of Mr Chan demonstrates how medical professionals navigate these crucial conversations, highlighting the cultural, emotional, and practical challenges they face.

Case Study: Navigating End-of-Life Communication for Mr Chan

Mr Chan, a 68-year-old retired teacher, was diagnosed with advanced lung cancer two years ago. Despite undergoing several rounds of chemotherapy, his condition had progressively worsened, and his recent imaging results showed widespread metastasis. Upon his latest hospital admission, his healthcare team, led by Dr Lee, recognized that Mr Chan's illness was no longer responsive to treatment and that his prognosis was limited. In light of these developments, Dr Lee decided it was crucial to engage in an end-of-life (EOL) conversation with Mr Chan and his family. The primary aim was to discuss Mr Chan's health condition, explore his treatment options, and understand his preferences for care. Dr Lee arranged a family meeting, bringing together Mr Chan, his wife, and their two adult children in a private consultation room.

During the meeting, Dr Lee carefully explained Mr Chan's current health status, emphasizing that while aggressive treatments such as chemotherapy were still an option, these might not provide significant benefit at this stage. Instead, she introduced the option of transitioning to palliative care, focusing on symptom management and improving his quality of life in his remaining time. She also broached sensitive topics, such as Mr Chan's preferences for resuscitation and whether he would prefer to receive care at home or in the hospital. Mr Chan expressed a strong preference to avoid further invasive treatments, stating that he valued spending time with his family and wished to remain at home. He shared that his priority was comfort and quality of life rather than prolonging life through aggressive measures. However, his family, particularly his eldest son, found this decision difficult to accept. His son expressed concerns about how they could manage Mr Chan's symptoms at home and whether they were fully aware of all possible medical interventions.

To address the family's concerns, Dr Lee provided detailed information about the support available through palliative care services, including at-home nursing visits, pain management, and emotional and psychological support for both Mr Chan and his family members. She also emphasized that transitioning to palliative care did not mean giving up but rather ensuring that Mr Chan's remaining time was spent according to his wishes. With the support and clarity provided by Dr Lee, Mr Chan's family gradually accepted his decision. They expressed relief knowing that Mr Chan would be surrounded by loved ones in a comfortable and familiar environment. Dr Lee then coordinated with the hospital's palliative care team to set up the necessary services and follow-up visits at Mr Chan's home. The above case study illustrates the complexity and sensitivity of EOL communication in clinical practice. It highlights how healthcare professionals, by engaging in open, honest, and culturally sensitive conversations, can align care decisions with the patient's values and preferences while also addressing the emotional needs of the family.

The above case study reflects these EOL conversations often encompass sensitive topics, including the likely progression of illness, pain management, resuscitation preferences, palliative care, and the patient's desires regarding quality versus quantity of life. EOL communication is essential for aligning medical care with patients' values and ensuring that decisions are made collaboratively (Blackhall et al., 2014; Puntillo & McAdam, 2006). It also helps to provide emotional and psychological support, reduce anxiety, and promote a sense of dignity for patients as they face the final stage of their lives. By engaging in these conversations, medical professionals can build trust with patients and their families, ensuring that care is compassionate, respectful, and tailored to meet the patient's individual needs and cultural values.

The Feature of EOL in Chinese Context

In Western healthcare systems, however, unlike the Chinese context, there is a strong emphasis on patient autonomy, where patients are encouraged to actively participate in decision-making about their own care (Houska & Loučka, 2019). This is often facilitated through mechanisms like advance directives (ADs) and advance care planning (ACP), which allow individuals to document their preferences for future medical care and ensure that their wishes are respected even when they may no longer be able to communicate them directly (Emanuel et al., 1991). For example, an elderly patient with a chronic illness might complete an advance directive specifying that they do not want to be placed on life support if their condition becomes critical, ensuring their preference is honoured even if they become unconscious or unable to communicate. These frameworks promote transparency and informed decision-making, empowering patients to retain control over their healthcare journey (Svendsen et al., 2024). However, in Hong Kong, where Chinese cultural values such as filial piety, collectivism, and a deep respect for authority are prevalent, the approach to EOL communication is markedly different (Pun et al., 2018). The concept of death remains a sensitive and taboo subject in Chinese culture, leading to hesitancy among both healthcare professionals and families to engage in open discussions about EOL issues (Pun, 2022; Pun et al., 2020). Conversations about death are often seen as bringing bad luck or causing emotional distress, which can complicate efforts to discuss prognosis and treatment preferences openly (Goldsteen et al., 2006). For instance, a doctor may find it challenging to discuss a terminal diagnosis with a patient's family, as they might believe that openly talking about death could worsen the patient's condition or bring misfortune to the family.

In Hong Kong's healthcare context, family members frequently take a central role in medical decision-making, with many patients choosing to defer decisions to their children, spouses, or other relatives (Cherry, 2015). For example, in Hong Kong, a doctor treating an elderly patient with advanced cancer might be approached by the patient's children or main carer, who insist that the doctor not disclose the severity of the illness directly to their parent or the patient's partner, believing that this information could cause undue distress and worsen their health. This reflects the cultural value of collectivism, where the family unit is prioritized over individual autonomy. Such emphasis on collectivism means that health-related decisions, in the Chinese context, are often viewed as a shared responsibility among family members, who work together to protect the well-being and emotional state of their loved one, sometimes even overriding the patient's own right to be fully informed.

In addition, it is common for families to request that clinicians withhold certain information, such as a terminal prognosis, from the patient, in an effort to protect them from emotional harm or to maintain hope

(Pun et al., 2023). This practice is rooted in the cultural belief that maintaining positivity can influence health outcomes and that confronting a terminal diagnosis too directly may lead to unnecessary suffering. As a result, clinicians, especially those working in the areas of primary care, or palliative care settings or maintaining a close therapeutic relationship with a patient, in Hong Kong face significant barriers when attempting to implement Western models of EOL communication, which typically prioritize transparency and patient autonomy. They should navigate complex family dynamics and cultural expectations during the communication with patient and family members while striving to provide patient-centred care (Srivastava, 2014). Healthcare professionals should, in these conversations, carefully balance respecting the family's wishes and cultural norms with their duty to prioritize the patient's well-being, autonomy, and right to be informed, often requiring sensitive negotiation and culturally appropriate communication strategies. Such cultural divergence creates ethical dilemmas for healthcare professionals who must balance respecting the family's wishes with their professional obligation to keep the patient fully informed (Mitnick et al., 2010). Therefore, effective EOL communication in Hong Kong requires a culturally sensitive approach that acknowledges these values and seeks to build trust with both the patient and their family members (Pun et al., 2018). This approach involves negotiating with families, providing them with education on the importance of open communication, and exploring culturally appropriate ways to engage patients in these difficult conversations. The next section will outline the ongoing challenges and priorities in teaching end-of-life communication within the Hong Kong context, focusing on the need for culturally sensitive approaches and the development of effective strategies to prepare medical professionals for these complex interactions.

Teaching End-of-Life Communication: Challenges and Priorities

Cultural Sensitivity

One perhaps can navigate the complex interplay between respecting cultural values and fulfilling their ethical obligation to provide clear and compassionate communication. In the Hong Kong context, traditional Chinese values such as filial piety, collectivism, and the taboo around discussing death heavily influence how end-of-life (EOL) conversations are conducted (Pun et al., 2018). For instance, clinicians may encounter families who prefer not to disclose a terminal prognosis to the patient, believing that such information could harm the patient's emotional state or worsen their condition. This cultural belief is rooted in the idea that positivity and maintaining hope can have a therapeutic effect on health outcomes (Pun et al., 2023).

An example commonly observed in the Hong Kong hospital context is a medical student witnessing a consultation in a geriatric day ward where an elderly patient with advanced lung cancer is unaware of the true severity of their illness. During the consultation, the patient's family requests that the doctor avoid telling the patient about the terminal nature of the disease. They believe that such news could cause the patient significant emotional distress and potentially worsen their condition. Instead, they ask the doctor to focus on symptom management and to offer a more hopeful outlook. Respecting the family's wishes, the doctor chooses to present the information in a way that emphasizes symptom control and quality of life, while carefully assessing the patient's reactions to determine if they are ready for more information. The medical student learns that in these scenarios, doctors must navigate the delicate balance between respecting cultural values—such as the family's protective instincts—and fulfilling their ethical responsibility to provide compassionate and honest communication, all the while ensuring that the patient's well-being remains the priority.

With the above case scenario, one would learn that how to handle these sensitive situations requires a deep understanding of the cultural context and the use of specific communication strategies that align with Chinese values while ensuring ethical obligations are met (Pun et al., 2018). For example, doctors might be trained in techniques such as 'soft disclosure,' where information is gradually shared in a way that respects the patient's and family's cultural beliefs (Walczak et al., 2015). To illustrate the concept of "soft disclosure," a doctor might start the conversation by saying, "The recent test results have indicated some areas of concern in your lungs that we need to monitor closely," and then, over the course of several consultations, gradually disclose more details about the seriousness of the condition, allowing the patient and family time to absorb and process the information. This could involve first gauging the family's and patient's readiness to discuss the prognosis and then slowly introducing the conversation by framing it in a culturally appropriate manner.

In this soft approach to disclosing a patient's latest condition, the doctor can gradually steer the conversation to gauge the patient's openness to receiving more detailed information about their prognosis, while ensuring the discussion aligns with the patient's cultural and emotional readiness. Educators can perhaps use role-playing scenarios to help students practice navigating these delicate situations, ensuring that they develop the skills needed to balance cultural sensitivity with ethical patient care. For instance, educators might set up a role-playing exercise where a student acts as a doctor delivering difficult news to a simulated patient and their family, allowing the student to practice balancing the family's desire to withhold information with the ethical need to keep the patient informed, all the while using culturally appropriate language and techniques (see more from Pun, 2021a, 2021b).

The Role of Family in Decision-Making

In Hong Kong, family involvement in EOL conversations is not just common; it is expected, and the cultural norm is for families to play a central role in medical decision-making (Pun et al., 2023). The influence of "filial piety"—a Confucian value where children are expected to care for and make decisions on behalf of their aging parents—is deeply embedded in Hong Kong's healthcare context (Chan et al., 2012). This often results in situations where patients defer to their family members, typically their children, for decisions about their care. For example, in Hong Kong, an elderly patient diagnosed with a serious illness might say to their doctor, "I'll leave the decision to my children; they know what's best for me," reflecting the common practice of deferring medical decisions to family members in accordance with cultural expectations of filial duty in the Chinese context.

Medical students perhaps should be given communication training in managing family dynamics and understanding when it is appropriate to engage family members in decision-making. This includes developing strategies for navigating "collusion," a practice where families may ask clinicians to withhold critical information from the patient, believing it is in the patient's best interest (Chaturvedi et al., 2009; The et al., 2001). For example, a doctor may need to skilfully navigate a conversation where a family insists on avoiding any mention of a terminal diagnosis to preserve the patient's morale and sense of hope. To prepare students for these situations, training programmes can incorporate case studies and simulated role-plays where students practice negotiating with families, explaining the importance of patient autonomy, and exploring ways to involve the patient in decision-making without disregarding the family's wishes (Weiner & Cole, 2004; Kottewar et al., 2014). For example, in a training session, medical students might participate in a role-play where they practice explaining to a patient's family the importance of patient autonomy, while also finding a compromise that allows the patient to be involved in decision-making without undermining the family's desire to protect them. In some cases, this might mean finding compromises where a healthcare provider educates the family about the benefits of open communication and gradually involves the patient in discussions, ensuring that the patient's preferences are ultimately respected (Drossman et al., 2021).

Timing and Approach to EOL Conversations

One of the most significant challenges in EOL communication is determining the right time to initiate these conversations. In the context of EOL communication, "timing" refers to the careful and strategic selection of the most appropriate moment to initiate discussions about a patient's prognosis, treatment options, and end-of-life preferences (Bodi et al., 2022). This involves considering the patient's physical condition, emotional readiness, and cultural or family dynamics to ensure that the conversation is both sensitive and effective, minimizing discomfort and resistance from patients and their families. In Hong Kong, the timing and approach must be handled with great care, as both patients and families may feel uncomfortable discussing death-related topics (Pun et al., 2023). Medical students can recognize when patients and their families are emotionally and psychologically ready to discuss EOL matters and how to approach the topic in a culturally sensitive and compassionate manner. For example, a doctor might first build rapport with the patient and family over several visits, gradually assessing their emotional state and readiness, before gently introducing the topic by asking, "Have you and your family had a chance to think about your wishes for future care, should your condition change?"

Research shows that these conversations often happen too late, leaving patients and families unprepared for the final stages of life (Zakhour et al., 2015). For example, it is not uncommon for doctors to wait until the patient's condition deteriorates significantly before discussing EOL options, which can result in rushed decisions and increased distress for both the patient and their family members (Izumi & Van Son, 2016). Educators perhaps can emphasize the importance of initiating EOL discussions early, ideally before the patient's condition becomes critical, so that the patient and family have ample time to process the information and make informed decisions. To facilitate this, medical students can be trained using structured communication models like the SPIKES protocol, which offers a step-by-step approach for breaking bad news and managing difficult conversations (Baile et al., 2000). The SPIKES model includes six stages: *Setting up the interview*, where the doctor prepares the environment and ensures privacy; *Perception of the patient*, which involves assessing the patient's understanding of their situation; *Invitation from the patient*, where the doctor gauges how much information the patient wishes to receive; *Knowledge sharing*, where the doctor delivers the information in clear, straightforward language; *Emotions and empathetic response*, which focuses on addressing the patient's emotional reaction with compassion; and finally, *Summarize and strategize*, where the doctor summarizes the discussion and collaborates with the patient on the next steps and care plan. Educators may also present examples where clinicians used this approach effectively, demonstrating how timely and structured EOL conversations can lead to better patient outcomes and a smoother transition to palliative care (Steinberg & Fratkin, 2021). This can be reinforced through simulation exercises that allow students to practice timing their conversations appropriately and using culturally respectful language to engage patients and families in these important discussions.

Integrating Western and Chinese Communication Models

To enhance patients' clinical outcomes, especially during the EOL context, Hong Kong's healthcare system should move beyond the simple adoption of Western communication models and develop a culturally appropriate framework that integrates both Western and Chinese communication practices (Pun et al., 2018). Commonly used in Western medical education, models such as the Calgary-Cambridge guide and the SPIKES protocol focus on teaching communication skills centred on patient care, open dialogue, and empathy. However, the direct and individual-focused nature of these models may conflict with Hong Kong's cultural norms, which prioritize family involvement and often aim to protect patients from distressing information (Pun et al., 2021). In contrast, Chinese communication practices in healthcare are more hierarchical and family-oriented, with an emphasis on maintaining harmony and minimizing conflict. These values are evident in the way sensitive topics like death and terminal illness are handled, as families often prefer to manage these conversations to shield patients from emotional distress. To be effective, a culturally adapted communication model for Hong Kong should incorporate these values while ensuring that patients receive the necessary information to make informed healthcare decisions (see more from Pun et al., 2020). A hybrid communication model that merges the structured, patient-centred approach of Western models with the cultural sensitivity of Chinese practices could be particularly effective in this context (Pun et al., 2018). Such a model would train medical students to communicate clearly and empathetically with both patients and their families, while respecting cultural values, family dynamics, and preferences. This balanced approach would help create a framework that supports both patient autonomy and the cultural context in which healthcare decisions are made (Pun et al., 2020).

Training Methods for Teaching Clinical Communication

Training methods for teaching clinical communication in Hong Kong include several effective approaches tailored to the local context (Pun, 2023). One of the most impactful methods perhaps is the use of simulated patient encounters (Smith et al., 2018). These simulations provide students with a controlled environment where they can practice their communication skills, receive direct feedback from instructors, and learn to navigate complex cultural dynamics. In EOL scenarios, simulations can be designed to include interactions with family members, allowing students to practice engaging with both the patient and their family (Pun et al., 2021, 2018). Another method is role-playing with real cases, where incorporating actual case studies from local hospitals helps students understand the nuances of EOL communication specific to Hong Kong. By role-playing based on these real-life cases, students are exposed to the challenges they may encounter in their future practice, and they develop the flexibility needed to adapt Western communication models to fit the local cultural context (Pun et al., 2021). Additionally, multidisciplinary teaching is crucial, as the complexity of EOL communication requires input from various fields. Collaboration between medical educators, communication experts, and cultural specialists can provide students with a more comprehensive understanding of the communication challenges they will face in clinical settings, ensuring a well-rounded education that prepares them for real-world interactions (Pun et al., 2021).

In conclusion, as Hong Kong's healthcare system continues to evolve, there is a growing need for culturally sensitive clinical communication training, particularly for end-of-life (EOL) care. Medical students must be equipped with the skills to navigate the complexities of EOL communication within a culturally diverse society. By integrating Western communication models with Chinese cultural values, educators can better prepare students to deliver compassionate, patient-centred care that aligns with Hong Kong's unique cultural context. Developing a hybrid communication framework for EOL discussions not only enhances the quality of care for patients but also strengthens the therapeutic relationship between clinicians, patients, and their families. This approach ensures that medical students are well-prepared to meet the communication needs of their patients, fostering a more compassionate and culturally sensitive healthcare system that improves patient outcomes and supports both patient autonomy and family involvement.

References

Anselm, A. H., Palda, V., Guest, C. B., McLean, R. F., Vachon, M. L., Kelner, M., & Lam-McCulloch, J. (2005). Barriers to communication regarding end-of-life care: Perspectives of care providers. *Journal of Critical Care, 20*(3), 214–223.

Baile, W. F., Buckman, R., Lenzi, R., Glober, G., Beale, E. A., & Kudelka, A. P. (2000). SPIKES—A six-step protocol for delivering bad news: Application to the patient with cancer. *The Oncologist, 5*(4), 302–311.

Blackhall, L. J., Erickson, J., Brashers, V., Owen, J., & Thomas, S. (2014). Development and validation of a collaborative behaviors objective assessment tool for end-of-life communication. *Journal of Palliative Medicine, 17*(1), 68–74.

Bodi, S., Matus, C., & Hickey, D. (2022). Right place, right time: Facilitating end-of-life conversations. *The Journal of Family Practice, 71*(2), 74.

Chan, C. L., Ho, A. H., Leung, P. P., Chochinov, H. M., Neimeyer, R. A., Pang, S. M., & Tse, D. M. (2012). The blessings and the curses of filial piety on dignity at the end of life: Lived experience of Hong Kong Chinese adult children caregivers. *Journal of Ethnic and Cultural Diversity in Social Work, 21*(4), 277–296.

Chaturvedi, S. K., Loiselle, C. G., & Chandra, P. S. (2009). Communication with relatives and collusion in palliative care: A cross-cultural perspective. *Indian Journal of Palliative Care, 15*(1), 2.

Cherry, M. J. (2015). Re-thinking the role of the family in medical decision-making. *Journal of Medicine and Philosophy, 40*(4), 451–472.

Drossman, D. A., Chang, L., Deutsch, J. K., Ford, A. C., Halpert, A., Kroenke, K., et al. (2021). A review of the evidence and recommendations on communication skills and the patient–provider relationship: A Rome foundation working team report. *Gastroenterology, 161*(5), 1670–1688.

Emanuel, L. L., Barry, M. J., Stoeckle, J. D., Ettelson, L. M., & Emanuel, E. J. (1991). Advance directives for medical care—A case for greater use. *New England Journal of Medicine, 324*(13), 889–895.

Goldsteen, M., Houtepen, R., Proot, I. M., Abu-Saad, H. H., Spreeuwenberg, C., & Widdershoven, G. (2006). What is a good death? Terminally ill patients dealing with normative expectations around death and dying. *Patient Education and Counseling, 64*(1–3), 378–386.

Houska, A., & Loučka, M. (2019). Patients' autonomy at the end of life: A critical review. *Journal of Pain and Symptom Management, 57*(4), 835–845.

Izumi, S. S., & Van Son, C. (2016). "I didn't know he was dying": Missed opportunities for making end-of-life care decisions for older family members. *Journal of Hospice & Palliative Nursing, 18*(1), 74–81.

Kottewar, S. A., Bearelly, D., Bearelly, S., Johnson, E. D., & Fleming, D. A. (2014). Residents' end-of-life training experience: A literature review of interventions. *Journal of Palliative Medicine, 17*(6), 725–732.

Mitnick, S., Leffler, C., Hood, V. L., & American College of Physicians Ethics, Professionalism and Human Rights Committee. (2010). Family caregivers, patients and physicians: Ethical guidance to optimize relationships. *Journal of General Internal Medicine, 25*, 255–260.

Pun, J. (2021a). A study of Chinese medical students' communication pattern in delivering bad news: An ethnographic discourse analysis approach. *BMC Medical Education, 21*(286), 1–10.

Pun, J. (2021b). Communication about advance directives and advance care planning in the East Asian context: A systematic review. *Oncology Nursing Forum, 49*(1), 58–70.

Pun, J. (2022). The priorities, challenges, and scope of clinical communication teaching perceived by clinicians from different disciplines: A Hong Kong case study. *BMC Primary Care, 22*(158), 1–16.

Pun, J. (2023). *The Role of Language in Eastern and Western Health Communication*. Routledge.

Pun, J., Chan, E. A., Wang, S., & Slade, D. (2018). Health professional-patient communication practices in East Asia: An integrative review of an emerging field of research and practice in Hong Kong, South Korea, Japan, Taiwan, and Mainland China. *Patient Education and Counseling, 101*(7), 1193–1206.

Pun, J., Cheung, K. M., Chow, C. H. J., & Chan, W. L. (2020). Chinese perspective on end-of-life communication: A systematic review. *BMJ Supportive & Palliative Care, 14*, e30.

Pun, J., Cheung, K. M., & Chow, C. H. J. (2021). A systematic review of teaching end of life communication: The priorities, the challenges and the scope. *BMJ Supportive & Palliative Care, 12*(4), 368–375.

Pun, J., Chow, J. C. H., Fok, L., & Cheung, K. M. (2023). The role of patients' family members in end-of-life communication: An integrative review. *BMJ Open, 13*(2), e067304, 1–12.

Puntillo, K. A., & McAdam, J. L. (2006). Communication between physicians and nurses as a target for improving end-of-life care in the intensive care unit: Challenges and opportunities for moving forward. *Critical Care Medicine, 34*(11), S332–S340.

Sinuff, T., Dodek, P., You, J. J., Barwich, D., Tayler, C., Downar, J., et al. (2015). Improving end-of-life communication and decision making: The development of a conceptual framework and quality indicators. *Journal of Pain and Symptom Management, 49*(6), 1070–1080.

Smith, M. B., Macieira, T. G., Bumbach, M. D., Garbutt, S. J., Citty, S. W., Stephen, A., et al. (2018). The use of simulation to teach nursing students and clinicians palliative care and end-of-life communication: A systematic review. *American Journal of Hospice and Palliative Medicine®, 35*(8), 1140–1154.

Srivastava, R. H. (2014). Culture, religion, and family-centred care. In *Paediatric Patient and Family-Centred Care: Ethical and Legal Issues* (pp. 57–77).

Steinberg, K., & Fratkin, M. (2021). Transitions in palliative and end-of-life care. In *Palliative and Serious Illness Patient Management for Physician Assistants* (p. 416).

Svendsen, S. J., Grov, E. K., & Staats, K. (2024). Patients' experiences with shared decision-making in home-based palliative care–navigation through major life decisions. *BMC Palliative Care, 23*(1), 101.

The, A. M., Hak, T., Koëter, G., & van der Wal, G. (2001). Collusion in doctor-patient communication about imminent death: An ethnographic study. *Western Journal of Medicine, 174*(4), 247.

Walczak, A., Henselmans, I., Tattersall, M. H., Clayton, J. M., Davidson, P. M., Young, J., et al. (2015). A qualitative analysis of responses to a question prompt list and prognosis and end-of-life care discussion prompts delivered in a communication support program. *Psycho-Oncology, 24*(3), 287–293.

Weiner, J. S., & Cole, S. A. (2004). ACare: A communication training program for shared decision making along a life-limiting illness. *Palliative & Supportive Care, 2*(3), 231–241.

Zakhour, M., LaBrant, L., Rimel, B. J., Walsh, C. S., Li, A. J., Karlan, B. Y., & Cass, I. (2015). Too much, too late: Aggressive measures and the timing of end of life care discussions in women with gynecologic malignancies. *Gynecologic Oncology, 138*(2), 383–387.

9

Navigating Communication in Traditional Chinese Medicine: Strategies, Challenges, and Pedagogical Implications

The Role of Traditional Chinese Medicine (TCM) in Hong Kong

Traditional Chinese Medicine (TCM) holds a unique and influential position within Hong Kong's healthcare system, serving as a bridge between Western and Chinese cultural values. This duality allows TCM to thrive in a region where traditional practices are deeply rooted, yet modern healthcare standards and expectations, often aligned with Western Medicine (WM), are increasingly influential (Chung et al., 2007; Ng et al., 2022; Sun et al., 2017). Over the last few decades, TCM's popularity has expanded not only in East Asia but also on a global scale, as patients and healthcare practitioners alike seek holistic and integrative approaches to health and well-being (Xu & Xia, 2019). Unlike Western Medicine, which often focuses on diagnosing and treating specific symptoms or diseases, TCM emphasizes the interconnectedness of the body, mind, and spirit (Leung, 2015). It views health as a dynamic balance between various elements and focuses on harmonizing these aspects to achieve overall well-being. This holistic approach considers not only the physical state of the patient but also psychological, emotional, and

J. Pun, *Exploring and Teaching Healthcare Communication*,
https://doi.org/10.1007/978-3-031-08675-5_9

lifestyle factors (Harvie et al., 2019). In Hong Kong, this practice is particularly prominent in primary care settings where TCM practitioners cultivate long-term relationships with patients. These sustained interactions enable practitioners to understand patients' health trajectories comprehensively, facilitating tailored and effective treatments that go beyond immediate physical symptoms (Pun & Chor, 2022; Pun, 2022; Pun et al., 2019). Such relationships form the backbone of patient-centred care, which is crucial for achieving positive health outcomes in TCM.

Traditional Chinese Medicine (TCM) occupies a distinct and influential role in Hong Kong's healthcare landscape that aligns with both cultural and modern healthcare expectations. This integration has been bolstered by the Hong Kong Special Administrative Region (HKSAR) government's policies to establish and regulate TCM practices, ensuring that it remains a crucial component of primary care services. Since the early 2000s, public TCM clinics have been developed, and universities such as The University of Hong Kong (HKU), The Chinese University of Hong Kong (CUHK), and The Hong Kong Baptist University (HKBU) now provide professional qualifications for TCM practitioners (Pun & Chor, 2022). Hong Kong's unique cultural heritage, shaped by its colonial past and Chinese traditions, has allowed TCM to thrive alongside Western Medicine (WM) (Chiu & Sze, 2021). This duality offers an opportunity for comparative analysis between these two medical paradigms, especially in how they navigate cross-cultural expectations and clinical practices. TCM practitioners often employ culturally sensitive communication strategies, recognizing the importance of maintaining rapport and meeting patients' expectations, which are influenced by both Chinese and Western values (Pun, 2022).

Globally, the popularity of TCM has expanded as it appeals to those seeking holistic and integrative health solutions (Adams et al., 2017). In Hong Kong, this approach is particularly evident in primary care, where TCM practitioners develop long-term relationships with their patients, enabling them to offer treatments that encompass physical, psychological, and social aspects of health (Pun & Wong, 2022). Unlike WM, which focuses primarily on diagnosing and treating specific symptoms through empirical evidence, TCM adopts a more holistic approach that sees health as a balance of various elements, such as Yin-Yang and the Five

Elements, and views disease as an imbalance influenced by both the body and its environment (Pun & Chor, 2022). In practice, TCM consultations involve a personalized and comprehensive assessment, known as the "four methods"—inspection, auscultation and olfaction, inquiry, and palpation. This method allows practitioners to evaluate the patient's overall health and balance, leading to a diagnosis that considers not only symptoms but also the patient's lifestyle, environment, and emotions (Tian et al., 2024). Such assessments facilitate in-depth discussions between practitioners and patients, where the latter are encouraged to share their experiences and concerns. These sustained and interactive consultations are integral to building a strong practitioner-patient relationship, promoting shared decision-making, and fostering trust, which are essential for effective patient-centred care (Pun et al., 2019). The continuity of care in TCM is also significant. Patients often visit the same practitioner repeatedly, allowing the development of a long-term therapeutic relationship (Chung et al., 2015). This ongoing interaction contrasts with WM's episodic nature, where patients may frequently see different doctors. The trust established in these sustained relationships contributes to patient satisfaction, adherence to treatment, and improved health outcomes. Studies have shown that elderly patients in Hong Kong, in particular, express higher levels of satisfaction with TCM practitioners than with WM doctors due to these long-term relationships and the personalized attention they receive (Chung et al., 2007, 2015; Lam et al., 2009).

Furthermore, recent studies demonstrate the effectiveness of communication training programmes for TCM practitioners (Pun et al., 2019; Pun & Kong, 2023). These programmes aim to integrate conventional medical histories into TCM consultations, enhancing the practitioner's ability to understand the patient's full health trajectory and thus providing a more integrated and holistic treatment approach (Zhang & Chor, 2023). Such training helps TCM practitioners bridge the gap between conventional and traditional practices, promoting patient-centred care that respects cultural preferences while meeting modern medical standards (Zhang & Zhu, 2023). In summary, TCM's unique positioning in Hong Kong's healthcare system reflects its ability to bridge traditional Chinese values and modern Western healthcare standards. The holistic, patient-centred approach of TCM not only addresses physical symptoms but also considers patients' emotional and social needs, which are crucial for comprehensive health and well-being. This dual system enables TCM to play a vital role in Hong Kong's primary care settings, providing a model for integrative health practices that may be applied more broadly. The next section will further elaborate the nature of TCM communication in Hong Kong context.

The Nature of TCM Communication in Hong Kong

Traditional Chinese Medicine (TCM) is deeply rooted in Hong Kong's cultural and medical history, offering a unique blend of holistic practices that consider the patient's physical, emotional, and psychological well-being. People in Hong Kong welcome Traditional Chinese Medicine (TCM) because it aligns with their cultural beliefs and provides a personalized, holistic approach to health that integrates both preventive care and natural remedies. Many young adults in Hong Kong now turn to TCM for conditions like chronic pain, stress, and digestive issues, believing that its use of herbal remedies and acupuncture can restore balance and harmony in the body more naturally than Western medicine (Pun, 2021). This growing preference for TCM among the younger generation highlights a shift towards embracing traditional practices as a complement or alternative to conventional medical treatments. One possible reason to explain such popularity of TCM among Hong Kong population is because TCM practitioners focus on identifying imbalances in the body's energy systems—referred to as "Zheng"—through comprehensive diagnostics that include examining the pulse, life force, and organ functions (Pun, 2020; Pun et al., 2019). To do this, TCM practitioner may assess a patient's pulse and tongue appearance to determine energy blockages or deficiencies, guiding the use of herbal treatments or acupuncture to restore balance. This approach, distinct from Western Medicine (WM), emphasizes the interconnectedness of the body and its environment, taking into account the patient's lifestyle, diet, and emotional state as critical factors influencing health (Pun, 2020; Pun & Kong, 2023).

In Hong Kong, TCM consultations are typically conducted in Cantonese, and many patients prefer TCM, particularly for chronic conditions, due to the continuity of care and the trust developed through long-term relationships with practitioners (Pun, 2022). For example, an elderly patient with arthritis might choose to visit the same TCM practitioner for years, valuing the personalized treatment plans and the rapport built through consultations conducted in their native Cantonese. In most TCM consultation in Hong Kong context, one emphasizes a collaborative, patient-centred approach, engaging patients in discussions that explore their everyday experiences and habits to understand how these factors contribute to their health. During a consultation, a TCM practitioner may ask detailed questions about the patient's diet, sleep patterns, stress levels, and daily routines to collaboratively identify lifestyle factors that might be affecting their health and to tailor a treatment plan that fits their individual needs. This participatory approach encourages patients to share personal details, creating a more holistic and individualized treatment plan (Pun et al., 2019; Pun, 2020).

The diagnostic process in TCM includes four primary methods: inspection (observing the patient's physical appearance), auscultation and olfaction (listening and smelling), inquiry (asking detailed questions about symptoms and lifestyle), and palpation (feeling the pulse and other physical indicators). For instance, Mr Lee, a 45-year-old office worker in Hong Kong, visits a TCM clinic complaining of frequent headaches and digestive issues. The practitioner begins the diagnostic process with inspection, observing Mr Lee's complexion, tongue colour, and posture for signs of imbalance. Next, using auscultation and olfaction, the practitioner listens to the tone of his voice and takes note of any unusual body odours that might indicate underlying health issues. Following this, the practitioner conducts an inquiry, asking Mr Lee about his daily routines, dietary habits, stress levels, and sleep patterns to gather a comprehensive understanding of his symptoms and lifestyle. Finally, the practitioner performs palpation by feeling Mr Lee's pulse and pressing gently on his abdomen to detect any irregularities in his internal organs. Based on these observations, the practitioner identifies an imbalance in Mr Lee's energy system and recommends a tailored treatment plan, including acupuncture sessions and a customized herbal formula, to address the root causes of his symptoms. These methods collectively form a comprehensive assessment framework that enables TCM practitioners to evaluate a patient's condition holistically (Pun et al., 2019; Xutian et al., 2012). Unlike Western Medicine, which often relies heavily on technology and scientific data, TCM integrates personal and environmental factors, aiming to restore balance and harmony within the patient's body (Pun, 2020; Pun & Kong, 2023).

Research has shown that TCM consultations in Hong Kong prioritize building rapport through effective communication strategies, such as open-ended questioning and the use of discourse markers, which create space for patients to express their concerns freely (Pun et al., 2019; Pun & Chor, 2022; Pun, 2022). For an example, Ms Chan, a 38-year-old teacher, visits a TCM practitioner in Hong Kong for persistent fatigue and insomnia. During the consultation, the practitioner begins by asking open-ended questions like, "*Can you tell me more about how you've been feeling lately?*" and "*What do you think might be contributing to your sleeplessness?*" These questions allow Ms Chan to openly share her concerns and provide detailed information about her daily stressors and lifestyle. Throughout the conversation, the practitioner uses discourse markers such as "I understand" and "Go on" to show empathy and encourage her to continue expressing her thoughts. This approach not only builds trust but also helps Ms Chan feel heard and valued, allowing the practitioner to gather a fuller picture of her health situation. As a result, a personalized treatment plan is developed that takes into account her physical symptoms as well as the emotional and psychological factors influencing her well-being. Besides, TCM practitioners often employ small talk and personalized inquiries about the patient's lifestyle. For example, during a consultation, Mr Wong, a 55-year-old taxi driver, seeks treatment from a TCM practitioner for chronic back pain. The practitioner begins the session with small talk about Mr Wong's work routine and recent experiences on the road, creating a relaxed and friendly atmosphere. He then asks personalized questions about Mr Wong's daily habits, such as his posture during long hours of driving and his diet. These inquiries not only provide valuable insights into factors contributing to his back pain but also help build trust, making Mr Wong feel more comfortable and open to collaborating on a treatment plan. This approach of using small talk and personalized questions not only elicits important health information but also strengthens the practitioner-patient relationship, fostering trust and collaboration (Pun, 2020, 2022; Pun et al., 2019). This deep engagement allows TCM practitioners to maintain long-term therapeutic relationships, where patients return for follow-up consultations, reinforcing the continuity of care that is less common in WM settings (Pun et al., 2018, 2019). Such relationships have been shown to enhance patient satisfaction and compliance with treatment, as patients feel heard and involved in the decision-making process regarding their health (Pun & Kong, 2023).

The Role of Language in TCM Communication in Hong Kong

The role of language in TCM communication in Hong Kong is crucial for fostering effective, patient-centred care. In TCM consultations, rapport between practitioners and patients is built through active listening, shared decision-making, and holistic conversations that address both physical and emotional dimensions of health (Pun & Kong, 2023). TCM practitioners in Hong Kong incorporate a combination of verbal and non-verbal techniques to engage patients and establish a shared understanding of health conditions. For instance, a case study involving Ms Lau, a 60-year-old retiree with chronic knee pain, illustrates this approach. The practitioner starts with warm greetings and invites Ms Lau to sit comfortably, using non-verbal cues like eye contact and nodding to convey empathy and attentiveness. The practitioner then asks open-ended questions about her pain, daily routine, and emotional state, allowing Ms Lau to share her experiences in detail. By explaining the body's energy flow using simple analogies and gently palpating her knee for inflammation, the practitioner integrates both verbal and tactile communication methods. This comprehensive approach helps Ms Lau feel understood, creating a supportive environment conducive to collaboration and effective treatment. This culturally embedded communication style emphasizes continuity and collaboration, distinguishing TCM from Western Medicine (WM) by blending medical expertise with respect for patient autonomy and cultural context (Pun et al., 2018).

In their 2020 study, Pun and Chor explored the linguistic and communicative strategies of TCM practitioners in Hong Kong, specifically focusing on diagnostic interviews with chronic illness patients. Utilizing an ethnographic discourse analysis approach, the researchers recorded and analysed eight hours of Cantonese consultations involving 14 local patients at a university-operated clinic. The study revealed that TCM consultations often start with open-ended questions that give patients the freedom to express their symptoms and concerns. These questions range from general inquiries, such as "How have you been feeling lately?", to more specific biomedical and psychosocial questions, allowing practitioners to gain a comprehensive understanding of the patient's condition and integrate their lifestyle and environmental factors into diagnosis. The analysis further highlighted that TCM practitioners use both structured and informal questioning to explore patients' daily habits, including diet, sleep patterns, and stress levels, which are critical for creating personalized treatment plans. The use of sentence-final particles (SFPs) and discourse markers (DMs) was also observed, which helped practitioners manage conversations, demonstrate epistemic commitment, and establish common ground with patients. These linguistic elements play a vital role in promoting patient participation and treatment compliance by creating a supportive and cooperative environment. Overall, the study emphasized that such strategies are key to implementing a patient-centred approach, as personalized inquiries and small talk help strengthen the practitioner-patient relationship, fostering trust and collaboration. These findings provide insights into how TCM communication practices in Hong Kong incorporate verbal and non-verbal elements to achieve culturally embedded and effective patient care.

Another study by Pun (2020), who explores the interactional dynamics within Traditional Chinese Medicine (TCM) consultations in Hong Kong, focuses on the concept of "touch" as a holistic communication and diagnostic tool. The study uses ten hours of audio recordings from a university-operated TCM clinic, involving a registered practitioner and nine patients. Data were collected through these recordings and ethnographic observations, with transcripts analysed for patterns using discourse analysis. The findings reveal that TCM consultations incorporate multiple diagnostic methods, known as si-zhen (望, 闻, 问, 切)—observation, auscultation, inquiry, and palpation—to co-construct a comprehensive understanding of the patient's body condition. The study highlights the importance of these "touch" moments, both literal and metaphorical, in building rapport and ensuring patient-centred care. By explaining symptoms using culturally relevant terms and maintaining a dialogue that includes small talk and reassurance, practitioners create an environment conducive to shared decision-making and long-term relationships. The study emphasizes the need for communication skills training for TCM practitioners to improve clinical outcomes, patient satisfaction, and treatment adherence.

Pun and Kong (2023) extended this work by exploring how communication training can enhance TCM practitioners' skills, particularly in integrating conventional medical histories into TCM consultations. Highlighting the importance of bridging the communication gap between TCM and conventional medicine, they conducted a randomized control trial involving eight registered TCM practitioners in Hong Kong, divided into experimental and control groups. The experimental group received training based on the Calgary-Cambridge guide, adapted to the Hong Kong context, to enhance skills in discussing and incorporating conventional medical histories into TCM consultations.

The study utilized audio-recorded consultations at three stages: pre-training, immediately post-training, and three months post-training, to assess the long-term effects of the training. Findings showed that practitioners who received training significantly improved their patient-centred communication skills, with a noticeable increase in open-ended questions and more comprehensive incorporation of patients' conventional medical histories. This approach allowed for a more holistic understanding of patients' conditions, strengthening the practitioner-patient rapport. The study highlighted the effectiveness of personalized communication strategies, such as exploring patients' daily experiences, which fostered patient engagement and created a shared understanding in the treatment process.

Additionally, trained practitioners exhibited increased confidence and skill in discussing both TCM and conventional medical histories, facilitating a more integrated care approach. This method was crucial in making patients feel heard and supported, leading to higher levels of satisfaction and adherence to treatment plans. However, the study also noted that the benefits of the training diminished over time, indicating a need for continuous professional development and refresher courses to maintain improved communication skills.

The research demonstrates the importance of integrating conventional medical history into TCM consultations for a comprehensive, patient-centred approach.

Another study is by Pun (2022), who investigates the role of Traditional Chinese Medicine (TCM) consultations in Hong Kong in fostering patient-centred care for elderly patients, using the Community of Practice (CoP) framework. The study employed ethnographic and inductive qualitative discourse analysis, observing interactions between a Cantonese-speaking TCM practitioner and ten elderly patients with chronic illnesses. Data were collected through audio recordings, which were then transcribed and analysed to identify communication patterns. The findings reveal that TCM practitioners use open-ended questions, personalized inquiries, and culturally relevant language to engage patients actively, promoting a collaborative environment where patients feel empowered to participate in their treatment. The study highlights the use of small talk and TCM-specific terminology to build rapport, manage uncertainty, and achieve consensus, ultimately enhancing patient satisfaction and adherence to treatment. The research emphasizes the need for TCM practitioners to develop effective communication skills to support holistic, patient-centred care, particularly for the elderly population. The above findings from the four studies in Hong Kong context emphasize the significance of effective communication training for TCM practitioners in Hong Kong, highlighting how a patient-centred, culturally sensitive approach can bridge the gap between traditional and conventional medical practices, ultimately enhancing patient outcomes and satisfaction.

Establishing rapport in TCM consultations is fundamental and unique, forming a cornerstone of effective patient care. Studies have shown that TCM practitioners in Hong Kong excel at cultivating close, trusting relationships with their patients through ongoing consultations and open dialogue. This process is characterized by patient-centred care, where the practitioners address not only the physical symptoms but also the emotional and psychological needs of the patient (Pun et al., 2019). For example, a practitioner might engage a patient in a conversation about their emotional well-being and stress levels while discussing physical symptoms such as fatigue or digestive issues. This holistic approach allows the practitioner to create a comprehensive treatment plan that takes into account all aspects of the patient's life (Pun, 2022; Pun & Kong, 2023).

By viewing the patient as a whole person rather than focusing solely on their symptoms, TCM practitioners provide a more personalized and empathetic consultation experience. They may ask about a patient's lifestyle habits, such as their daily routine, diet, and sleep patterns, to understand how these factors influence their health. For instance, a practitioner might inquire about a patient's work-life balance and dietary habits to identify stressors or nutritional deficiencies contributing to their condition. The consistent use of open-ended questioning and active engagement helps patients understand their health conditions better and empowers them to participate in their own treatment. This participatory approach not only enhances patient satisfaction but also promotes adherence to treatment plans (Pun & Chor, 2022; Pun et al., 2019).

Communication Challenges in Teaching TCM

Teaching communication in TCM settings presents distinct challenges, especially when attempting to integrate communication models commonly used in Western Medicine (WM). For example, teaching communication in TCM settings might involve training practitioners to incorporate Western diagnostic information, such as explaining lab results or imaging findings, into TCM consultations while maintaining a holistic, patient-centred approach. Additionally, practitioners may be taught how to use open-ended questions and culturally sensitive language to bridge the gap between WM's data-driven methods and TCM's emphasis on subjective patient experiences (Dean et al., 2016; Pun & Kong, 2023). While both TCM and WM aim to provide effective patient care, their approaches differ significantly. WM tends to be data-driven, relying heavily on diagnostic tools, lab results, and empirical evidence. In contrast, TCM emphasizes subjective patient experiences and holistic diagnostics, which involve assessing the patient's energy flow, lifestyle, and emotional state. For example, WM may focus on imaging and blood tests to diagnose a musculoskeletal issue, while TCM might also consider the patient's stress levels, diet, and work posture as contributing factors (Pun et al., 2019). As a result, TCM practitioners provide a more comprehensive and individualized treatment plan that not only addresses the physical symptoms but also considers the patient's overall lifestyle and well-being, which may be overlooked by the purely diagnostic approach of WM. A recent study examined the effects of communication training for TCM practitioners to improve their ability to integrate patients' WM histories into TCM consultations (Pun & Kong, 2023). Practitioners trained in patient-centred communication techniques, like those from the Calgary-Cambridge model, were better able to merge the two approaches. For instance, they learned how to incorporate WM data, such as a patient's blood pressure history, into the TCM consultation, explaining how it aligns with or differs from TCM diagnostics. The training led to improved interactions, resulting in stronger rapport and higher patient satisfaction, as patients felt their entire medical history was considered in the consultation.

The findings from these studies offer practical insights for educators and researchers looking to develop communication curricula for TCM practitioners. Training programmes should emphasize developing questioning techniques, active listening skills, and the ability to explain complex medical concepts in an accessible manner. For example, TCM practitioners could be trained to ask questions that explore both physical symptoms and lifestyle factors, such as, "*Can you tell me about your typical daily diet?*" or "*How do you manage stress in your work environment?*" These questions encourage patients to share relevant information that aids in diagnosis and treatment planning (Pun, 2022; Pun et al., 2019). Interactive teaching methods, such as role-playing and simulated consultations, can help practitioners refine these skills in a controlled, supportive environment. For example, practitioners could participate in role-plays where they practice building rapport with simulated patients by exploring both their physical complaints and emotional concerns. Additionally, integrating cultural elements specific to Hong Kong—like understanding the importance of addressing patients' interpersonal concerns and building long-term relationships—can enhance communication training further. For instance, training sessions could include modules on how to use culturally appropriate language and non-verbal cues to foster trust and connection during consultations (Pun & Chor, 2022; Pun et al., 2018).

Conclusion

Traditional Chinese Medicine provides a holistic and culturally embedded framework for patient care in Hong Kong. By prioritizing the development of deep practitioner-patient relationships and addressing patients' emotional and psychological needs alongside their physical symptoms, TCM offers an alternative to the clinical, data-focused approach of Western Medicine. The studies discussed underscore the importance of effective communication in delivering high-quality TCM care and propose practical strategies for teaching and implementing these techniques in clinical practice. As Hong Kong's healthcare system evolves, integrating communication training that blends both TCM and WM principles will be crucial for ensuring patient satisfaction and improving overall health outcomes.

References

Adams, J., Andrews, G., & Barnes, J. (2017). *Traditional, Complementary and Integrative Medicine: An International Reader*. Bloomsbury Publishing.

Chiu, S. W., & Sze, T. O. (2021). Revival or innovation? Chinese medicine at the crossroads of professionalization in Hong Kong. *SSM-Qualitative Research in Health, 1*, 100004.

Chung, V., Wong, E., Woo, J., Vi Lo, S., & Griffiths, S. (2007). Use of traditional Chinese medicine in the Hong Kong Special Administrative Region of China. *The Journal of Alternative and Complementary Medicine, 13*(3), 361–368.

Chung, V. C., Yip, B. H., Griffiths, S. M., Yu, E. L., Liu, S., Ho, R. S., et al. (2015). Patients' experience of Chinese medicine primary care services: Implications on improving coordination and continuity of care. *Scientific Reports, 5*(1), 18853.

Dean, S. J., Zaslawski, C., Roche, M., & Adams, J. (2016). "Talk to Them": Teaching communication skills to students of traditional Chinese medicine. *Journal of Nursing Education and Practice.*

Harvie, A., Steel, A., & Wardle, J. (2019). Traditional Chinese medicine self-care and lifestyle medicine outside of Asia: A systematic literature review. *The Journal of Alternative and Complementary Medicine, 25*(8), 789–808.

Lam, Y. C., Cheng, C. W., Peng, H., Law, C. K., Huang, X., & Bian, Z. (2009). Cancer patients' attitudes towards Chinese medicine: A Hong Kong survey. *Chinese Medicine, 4*, 1–8.

Leung, B. (2015). *Traditional Chinese Medicine: The Human Dimension.* Routledge.

Ng, T. K., Lo, M. F., & Fong, B. Y. (2022). Knowledge, attitude, utilisation and satisfaction of traditional Chinese medicine in Hong Kong. *International Journal of Pharmaceutical and Healthcare Marketing, 16*(1), 123–137.

Pun, J., Chan, E. A., Wang, W., & Slade, D. (2018). Health professional–patient communication practices in East Asia: An integrative review of an emerging field of research and practice in Hong Kong, South Korea, Japan, Taiwan and Mainland China. *Patient Education and Counseling, 101*(7), 1195–1206. https://doi.org/10.1016/j.pec.2018.01.019

Pun, J. (2020). Moments of 'touch' as a way for mental support in Traditional Chinese Medicine consultations: Analysis of the interactional process of co-constructing understanding of the patient's body conditions in Hong Kong. *Complementary Therapies in Medicine, 52*, 102516.

Pun, J. (2021). A study of Chinese medical students' communication pattern in delivering bad news: An ethnographic discourse analysis approach. *BMC Medical Education, 21*(286), 1–10.

Pun, J. (2022). The active participation of elderly patients in traditional Chinese medicine consultations as means to creating a Community of Practice: A case study in Hong Kong. *Frontiers in Psychology, 13*, 948988.

Pun, J., & Chor, W. (2022). Use of questioning between traditional Chinese medicine practitioners and patients to realize TCM philosophy: Holism, five elements and Yin-Yang in the context of doctor–patient communication. *Health Communication, 37*(2), 163–176.

Pun, J., & Kong, B. C. K. (2023). An exploratory study of communication training for Chinese medicine practitioners in Hong Kong to integrate patients' conventional medical history. *BMC Complementary Medicine and Therapies, 23*(10), 1–16.

Pun, J., & Wong, W. (2022). Navigating communication between conventional medicine and traditional Chinese medicine: A case study of patients with cancer in Hong Kong. *Supportive Care in Cancer, 30*, 5729–5735.

Pun, J., Chor, W., & Zhong, L. (2019). Delivery of patient-centered care in complementary medicine: Insights and evidence from the Chinese medical practitioners and patients in primary care consultations in Hong Kong. *Complementary Therapies in Medicine, 45*, 198–204.

Sun, K. S., Cheng, Y. H., Wun, Y. T., & Lam, T. P. (2017). Choices between Chinese and Western medicine in Hong Kong–interactions of institutional environment, health beliefs and treatment outcomes. *Complementary Therapies in Clinical Practice, 28*, 70–74.

Tian, D., Chen, W., Xu, D., Xu, L., Xu, G., Guo, Y., & Yao, Y. (2024). A review of traditional Chinese medicine diagnosis using machine learning: Inspection, auscultation-olfaction, inquiry, and palpation. *Computers in Biology and Medicine, 170*, 108074.

Xu, J., & Xia, Z. (2019). Traditional Chinese Medicine (TCM)—Does its contemporary business booming and globalization really reconfirm its medical efficacy & safety? *Medicine in Drug Discovery, 1*, 100003.

Xutian, S., Cao, D., Wozniak, J., Junion, J., & Boisvert, J. (2012). Comprehension of the unique characteristics of traditional Chinese medicine. *The American Journal of Chinese Medicine, 40*(02), 231–244.

Zhang, C., & Chor, W. (2023). Realizing holism in traditional Chinese medicine (TCM) consultations through the voice of TCM (VOTCM): An interactional analytical approach. *Health Communication, 38*(2), 275–284.

Zhang, Z., & Zhu, M. (2023). Holistic view of TCM on cancer integrative therapy. *Future Integrative Medicine, 2*(3), 159–167.

10

Exploring Veterinary Medicine Communication in Bilingual Context

Veterinary Communication in Hong Kong

In Hong Kong, the development of effective communication skills in veterinary medicine is particularly crucial due to the city's unique linguistic and professional landscape. Despite the increasing demand for veterinary services, there has been limited research exploring the role of communication in this context (Pun, 2020). Language plays a fundamental role in veterinary communication, acting as the primary medium through which veterinarians, veterinary nurses, and pet owners exchange crucial information about animal health and care (Bard et al., 2017). A veterinarian might need to explain the details of a surgical procedure and post-operative care to a pet owner or carer, ensuring that the client understands how to administer medication, monitor the pet's recovery, and recognize signs of complications—all of which require clear and accurate communication. In veterinary practice, effective communication is important because it goes beyond simply explaining medical procedures; it involves building rapport, fostering trust, and ensuring that clients fully understand the health status and needs of their pets (Coe et al., 2008). A veterinarian might take time to listen to a pet owner's concerns,

J. Pun, *Exploring and Teaching Healthcare Communication*,
https://doi.org/10.1007/978-3-031-08675-5_10

answer questions patiently, and provide reassurance, thereby building trust and ensuring that the owner feels confident and well-informed about their pet's treatment plan and overall health. This is particularly important in the context of veterinary medicine in Hong Kong, where language barriers frequently arise between English-speaking veterinarians and Cantonese-speaking clients (Pun, 2020). For example, an English-speaking veterinarian may struggle to explain the symptoms and treatment options for a pet's illness to a Cantonese-speaking client, who may not fully grasp the medical terminology or instructions given, potentially leading to misunderstandings or non-compliance with the prescribed care. Misunderstandings or miscommunications can lead to client dissatisfaction, improper care, or even negative health outcomes for pets (Adams & Frankel, 2007). If a veterinarian's explanation of a medication schedule is not clearly understood by the pet owner due to a language barrier, the owner might administer the medication incorrectly, potentially resulting in the pet's condition worsening or not improving as expected. Therefore, the ability to communicate clearly and compassionately in a language that pet owners understand is not just a professional skill but a critical component of effective veterinary practice (Bonvicini & Keller, 2006; Kogan et al., 2021). This skill goes beyond merely exchanging information; it requires veterinarians to simplify complex medical terms and convey them in an accessible way, ensuring that pet owners fully comprehend their pet's condition, treatment options, and care instructions. Such clarity not only builds trust but also fosters cooperation, increasing the likelihood that pet owners will follow medical advice, ultimately leading to better outcomes for animals (Adams & Kurtz, 2006). By creating a supportive and collaborative environment, veterinarians can strengthen the veterinarian-client relationship, manage expectations effectively, and reduce potential misunderstandings or conflicts (Shaw & Coe, 2024). Therefore, communicating in a clear and compassionate manner is indispensable for successful veterinary practice, as it directly influences both client trust and the overall quality of animal care (Englar et al., 2016). Given these challenges, it becomes essential to explore how veterinary professionals can be better equipped with bilingual communication skills and strategies tailored to Hong Kong's unique linguistic and cultural environment (Pun, 2020, 2021). This chapter investigates these complexities, highlighting the need for pedagogical approaches that align with the demands of practice in the region. This chapter investigates the complexities of veterinary communication in Hong Kong, where bilingual communication skills are vital but often underdeveloped in formal veterinary training. Drawing on recent studies, this chapter offers insights into how pedagogical approaches can be adapted to better prepare veterinary professionals for the linguistic and cultural realities of practice in Hong Kong.

Communication Skills in Veterinary Practice

Effective communication in veterinary practice is integral for achieving positive outcomes in patient care. Communication in this field often involves difficult discussions with clients, such as addressing terminal diagnoses, treatment failures, or euthanasia. Here, empathy and clear communication are essential to help clients make informed decisions while managing emotional responses (Dawson, 2010; Morris, 2012). For an example, Dr Chan, a veterinarian in Hong Kong, faced a challenging conversation with Mrs Wong, whose elderly Golden Retriever, Max, had been diagnosed with an aggressive form of cancer. After explaining the diagnosis in clear terms, Dr Chan discussed the possible treatment options. She balanced technical explanations with empathetic language, acknowledging the emotional toll on Mrs Wong. Given Max's age and the severity of the illness, Dr Chan gently introduced the option of palliative care to manage Max's pain and maximize his comfort. Dr Chan paused frequently, using open-ended questions like, "*How do you feel about Max's current quality of life?*" and "*What would be most important to you for Max in the time he has left?*" Mrs Wong expressed her concern about Max suffering and her fear of making the "Wrong" decision. Dr Chan reassured her, explaining that the decision to consider euthanasia, if needed, was about ensuring a peaceful transition for Max. Throughout, Dr Chan maintained eye contact and listened attentively to Mrs Wong's concerns, which helped Mrs Wong feel understood and supported during this difficult time. This example underscores how compassionate, clear communication can guide pet owners through challenging decisions, fostering trust and emotional support during some of the most difficult moments in veterinary care (Shaw & Lagoni, 2007).

Research highlights that when veterinarians employ client-centred communication strategies—such as using open-ended questions, non-verbal cues, and empathetic language—clients report higher satisfaction and adherence to treatment recommendations (see more from Adams & Kurtz, 2006; Pun, 2020). For instance, a veterinarian discussing a complex treatment plan with a client might use open-ended questions like, "*What are your main concerns about this treatment for Bella?*" or "*How comfortable do you feel with the next steps?*" Alongside maintaining eye contact and nodding to show attentiveness, these techniques help the client feel heard and respected, leading to greater trust in the veterinarian's recommendations and a stronger commitment to the treatment plan (McCracken, 2016). These skills also mitigate potential misunderstandings, which are especially critical in cases of terminal illness and other sensitive topics (Pun, 2021, 2023). In addition to client interactions, veterinary practice requires precise communication within interdisciplinary teams (Han et al., 2024). For example, during a handover in a veterinary hospital, a veterinarian might clearly outline a patient's condition, recent treatments, and any specific care instructions to the incoming team, ensuring continuity of care. By using precise language and confirming team members' understanding, the veterinarian helps prevent miscommunication, which is crucial in a high-stakes, multidisciplinary environment. Veterinary professionals need to effectively relay information during handovers and consultations with other healthcare providers (Currie & White, 2012). Clear and concise language during medical handovers ensures the accurate transfer of vital information and contributes to the continuity of care across shifts and departments (Pun, 2021). Otherwise, miscommunications in these instances can lead to errors and suboptimal patient care.

The Role of English in Hong Kong Veterinary Medical Training

In veterinary education, communication is increasingly recognized as a crucial clinical skill, particularly in supporting client-centred care. Research has shown that clients value veterinarians who exhibit empathy, build rapport, and actively engage them in shared decision-making (Adams & Kurtz, 2006). These competencies foster a sense of support and respect, which in turn enhances client engagement and adherence to treatment recommendations (Adams & Kurtz, 2012). For veterinary students in Hong Kong, communication skills are especially vital due to the multilingual and multicultural landscape they must navigate (Pun, 2021). Training programmes need to address these demands by equipping students to balance technical explanations with accessible language and adapt communication to meet diverse client expectations (Scalese & Issenberg, 2005). For example, a veterinary student in Hong Kong may be consulting with an older Chinese client about her dog's chronic heart condition. Recognizing that the client may feel more comfortable with a straightforward and culturally sensitive approach, the student could describe the treatment plan in accessible language, using terms like "helping the heart work better" instead of complex medical jargon. Additionally, the student might respectfully consider the client's cultural values by discussing the treatment in a way that emphasizes family well-being and the pet's comfort, thus aligning the communication style with the client's expectations and cultural context. By developing these communication skills, veterinary graduates in Hong Kong will be better prepared to navigate the linguistic and cultural complexities of their field, ultimately fostering stronger client relationships and improving the quality of care in a diverse, multicultural society (Pun, 2020). This skillset is essential in Hong Kong's bilingual environment, where both English and Cantonese are commonly interwoven within clinical interactions.

English plays a prominent role in veterinary education in Hong Kong, as most textbooks, research publications, and academic resources are in English. Veterinary students are thus expected to attain high English proficiency for success in both their studies and clinical practice. However, studies reveal that students often encounter challenges with the academic and professional English required for their training (see more from the review study by Pun, 2020). For example, difficulties in understanding technical terminology, writing reports, and conveying complex diagnoses in English underscore the need for curriculum reforms that emphasize English for Specific Purposes (ESP) to meet the unique language requirements of veterinary medicine (Pun, 2021). Moreover, there is an increasing recognition that veterinary students must master disciplinary literacies—the genres, discourses, and communication strategies specific to their field. This includes the ability to interpret scientific texts, compose medical reports, and communicate effectively with clients and colleagues in both written and spoken formats (Pun & Onder-Ozdemir, 2023). Mastery of these skills is essential for students to meet the demands of their future careers in Hong Kong's multilingual veterinary sector. In practice, Hong Kong's veterinary professionals face added linguistic complexity in bilingual clinical settings, where practitioners frequently switch between Cantonese and English. This code-switching can complicate clinical exchanges, particularly when discussing complex medical terms or addressing sensitive topics with clients. Language barriers are further compounded by cultural expectations, underscoring the importance of cultural competence and the ability to navigate multilingual environments effectively (Pun, 2023).Thus, effective veterinary communication goes beyond technical knowledge. It requires cultural sensitivity, strong interpersonal skills, and linguistic flexibility to adapt language according to clients' preferences and needs. This adaptability is crucial for building rapport and establishing trust, which are foundational to effective client-centred care (Pun, 2020, 2021). Given these complexities, Hong Kong's bilingual environment offers a distinctive backdrop for understanding and refining veterinary communication practices, highlighting the need for adaptable strategies that align with the city's unique linguistic and cultural dynamics.

Veterinary Medicine Communication in Hong Kong

The bilingual context in Hong Kong provides a unique environment for exploring veterinary medicine communication due to its distinctive linguistic and cultural features. This environment is shaped by the coexistence of Cantonese and English, as well as Hong Kong's current status as a Special Administrative Region of China. This dual language setting creates both linguistic challenges and opportunities for veterinary communication, distinguishing it from other cultural contexts (see more from Pun, 2021). Veterinary practitioners in Hong Kong are often trained overseas in English-speaking countries, where the medium of instruction is predominantly English (Pun, 2020). The training does not typically prepare well for the bilingual realities they face upon returning to Hong Kong. While their medical terminology and clinical skills are developed in English, many of their clients, predominantly local pet owners, may have limited proficiency in English and prefer communication in Cantonese (Pun, 2021). For example, a veterinarian trained in Australia may be proficient in explaining medical procedures in English but struggle to communicate the same information effectively in Cantonese to local pet owners who are unfamiliar with English medical terminology. As a result, the veterinarian may rely heavily on veterinary nurses to translate complex terms and bridge the language gap, which can sometimes lead to miscommunication or misunderstandings if the nuances of the medical explanation are not fully conveyed in Cantonese. This gap necessitates the use of translanguaging practices (Li, 2018), where veterinarians and veterinary nurses switch between languages to ensure effective communication. Translanguaging has been observed as a natural and necessary strategy in clinical environments in Hong Kong, where bilingual staff navigate between English for professional terminology and Cantonese for client interactions (see more from Pun, 2021).

Moreover, the role of the veterinary nurse becomes essential in bridging this linguistic divide. Veterinary nurses often act as cultural and linguistic mediators, interpreting complex medical information and translating it into accessible language that resonates with local pet owners

(Almendros et al., 2024). Their role mirrors the practices seen in human healthcare settings in Hong Kong, where translanguaging is used to facilitate effective handover communication among hospital staff (Pun, 2021). This strategy is not just about language translation; it involves adjusting communication styles to fit cultural norms and expectations, ensuring that clients receive and understand information in a manner that aligns with their cultural background and linguistic proficiency. What's more, Hong Kong's multicultural nature adds another layer of complexity to veterinary communication (Pun, 2020). In addition to the predominant Cantonese-speaking population, there are expatriates and non-Cantonese-speaking Chinese residents, such as those from Mainland China who speak Putonghua. This requires veterinarians to be flexible and culturally competent, adapting their communication approach depending on the client's linguistic and cultural background. For example, a veterinarian might need to use Cantonese, English, and Mandarin in the same appointment to make sure three parties—veterinary nurse (Cantonese), local pet owner (Mandarin), and a domestic helper from Philippine or Indonesia (English)—all understand the diagnosis and treatment, while also being aware of their different cultural expectations. Unlike other regions where a single language may dominate veterinary practice, the Hong Kong context demands an ongoing negotiation of linguistic and cultural identities. This negotiation is reflected in the veterinary education curriculum and practice, emphasizing the need for veterinary students and practitioners to develop bilingual and bicultural communication skills (Pun, 2021). In short, Hong Kong's bilingual and multicultural setting, combined with the linguistic gaps between English-trained veterinarians and local clients, makes it a particularly rich context for exploring veterinary communication. This complex linguistic environment highlights the unique communication needs and challenges that veterinarians in Hong Kong face, particularly when managing sensitive conversations with diverse clients. Consequently, addressing these communication demands within veterinary education requires innovative teaching strategies, especially given the added pressure of balancing content-heavy coursework with the development of essential interpersonal skills.

Challenges in Teaching Veterinary Communication in Hong Kong

Teaching communication skills in veterinary programmes is often challenging due to the content-heavy nature of the curriculum. Students are expected to acquire extensive scientific knowledge alongside developing clinical communication skills (Pun, 2020, 2021). This often leaves little room for communication training, which can lead to gaps in students' preparedness for real-world clinical practice. One major challenge is the lack of alignment between the communication skills taught in academic settings and those required in clinical contexts. For example, while students may learn theoretical aspects of communication, they may not receive enough practical training in delivering difficult news or managing client relationships (Pun, 2020, 2021). Another challenge is the linguistic diversity in Hong Kong (Pun, 2023). Veterinary students often have to communicate with clients in Cantonese or English, and the switch between these languages can lead to communication breakdowns, particularly when discussing complex medical information (Pun & Onder-Ozdemir, 2023). To address these issues, veterinary programmes need to integrate more practical communication training that reflects the linguistic and cultural realities of veterinary practice in Hong Kong. To better prepare veterinary students for the communication demands of their profession, a more integrated and practical approach to teaching communication is needed. Drawing on insights from previous research (Pun, 2020, 2021, 2023), this section outlines a proposed curriculum that includes the following key components:

(a) **Multimodal Communication Training:** To address the diverse communication requirements in veterinary practice, students should be trained in multiple formats, including face-to-face consultations, written reports, and digital communication (Berrian et al., 2021). Practical exercises such as role-playing, case-based learning, and simulated client interactions can help students gain confidence and competence across various contexts. For instance, role-playing exercises allow students to practice verbal communication and empathy in a simulated client consultation, while case-based learning enables them to work through real-world scenarios, honing both their clinical and interpersonal skills. Additionally, simulated digital exchanges (such as email or text-based client inquiries) offer students a controlled environment to practice professionalism and clarity in written communication, an increasingly vital aspect of veterinary practice.

For example, in a Hong Kong veterinary programme, students could participate in a simulated consultation exercise where they are paired with an actor playing the role of a Cantonese-speaking pet owner who is anxious about her dog's recent diagnosis. The exercise begins with a role-play consultation in Cantonese, where students practice explaining the diagnosis in layman's terms, using culturally relevant expressions and demonstrating empathy to reassure the "client." After the consultation, students are tasked with writing a follow-up report in English, summarizing the case and documenting key details in professional medical language. Lastly, as part of a simulated digital communication module, students respond to a mock email from the client (in Cantonese), addressing her questions about the medication in a clear, respectful manner. By practicing these scenarios, students build competence across spoken, written, and digital formats, gaining confidence in how to adapt their communication style and language for both local clients and clinical documentation.

(b) **Client-Centred Communication:** Developing a client-centred approach is vital for effective veterinary practice, as building rapport and ensuring mutual understanding are central to client satisfaction and treatment adherence (Adams & Kurtz, 2006). Training programmes should emphasize skills such as empathy, active listening, and clarity in explanations. For example, students can practice explaining diagnoses and treatment plans in accessible language, ensuring clients grasp essential information about their pets' health. Empathy-building exercises, like reflective listening and feedback sessions, can further enhance students' ability to connect with clients, making them feel valued and respected. By fostering these interpersonal skills, students will be better prepared to create positive, trust-based relationships with clients.

For instance, in a training session focused on client-centred communication, vet students in Hong Kong might participate in an exercise where they engage with an actor portraying a Cantonese-speaking elderly pet owner who is very concerned about her dog's upcoming surgery. During the simulated consultation, students are encouraged to use active listening techniques, such as nodding, maintaining eye contact, and reflecting back the client's concerns to demonstrate understanding ("I understand you're worried about how the surgery will affect your dog's energy and health"). Students are then guided to practice explaining the surgery in simple, clear terms, perhaps using culturally familiar metaphors to reassure the client, such as comparing the procedure to a routine treatment. After the role-play, students receive feedback on their ability to convey empathy and clarity, as well as their skill in building rapport. Reflective exercises allow students to consider the emotional needs of clients in such situations, equipping them to respond sensitively and build trust, which is essential for fostering positive client relationships in real-world practice.

(c) **Cross-disciplinary Communication:** Veterinary professionals frequently collaborate with healthcare teams, including nurses, specialists, and administrative staff, making effective cross-disciplinary communication a critical skill (Han et al., 2024). Students should be trained to engage in clear, accurate information exchange during handovers and collaborative consultations, where details about a patient's condition, treatment history, and next steps must be effectively conveyed. Exercises such as interdisciplinary role-play or team-based scenarios can simulate real-life situations where students must collaborate and communicate effectively. This component of the curriculum will prepare students to work seamlessly with colleagues from different disciplines, ensuring continuity of care and enhancing the overall efficiency of veterinary services.

In a training exercise designed to build cross-disciplinary communication skills, veterinary students in Hong Kong might participate in a simulated team handover involving colleagues from various specialties, such as a veterinary nurse, a specialist surgeon, and an administrative assistant. The scenario could focus on a recent surgery performed on a dog with a complex medical history. The student is tasked with conveying critical details about the patient's condition in Cantonese, ensuring that each team member receives the relevant information in a clear and structured way. For example, the student would need to communicate to the nurse specific post-operative care steps, emphasize follow-up procedures with the administrative assistant for client scheduling, and consult with the surgeon regarding any necessary adjustments to the treatment plan. After the role-play, students receive feedback on their clarity, organization, and ability to tailor information to each team member's role. Through this exercise, they practice breaking down technical information into precise, accessible points, honing the skills necessary to work collaboratively and ensure consistent, high-quality patient care across a multilingual and multidisciplinary team.

(d) **Bilingual Communication Skills:** In Hong Kong's bilingual veterinary environment, the ability to switch fluently between English and Cantonese is an essential skill (Pun, 2020). Students should be trained to adapt their communication style according to the linguistic preferences of their clients, which may involve explaining complex medical terms in layman's language in both languages. Practical exercises, such as bilingual consultations with simulated clients, can help students practice language-switching fluidly while maintaining professionalism and clarity. Additionally, training in culturally sensitive communication will enable students to build rapport more effectively with clients, respecting their linguistic and cultural backgrounds. This bilingual skillset is crucial for veterinary practitioners in Hong Kong, allowing them to meet the diverse needs of their client base and enhance their service quality.

In a bilingual communication training session, veterinary students in Hong Kong could participate in a simulated consultation with an actor portraying a pet owner who prefers speaking in Cantonese but also understands some English medical terms. The student begins by explaining the pet's condition in Cantonese, using layman's terms to ensure comprehension, such as describing "heart disease" as "心臟問題" (heart issues) instead of complex medical terminology. As the consultation progresses, the actor (as the client) asks about specific terms they read in English online, like "cardiomyopathy," prompting the student to switch languages briefly to address the question in English before returning to Cantonese for the broader discussion.

After the exercise, students receive feedback on their ability to switch between languages smoothly and effectively, maintaining a clear, professional tone throughout. This practice helps students become more adept at adapting to the linguistic preferences of clients, ensuring that clients feel both understood and respected. By training in language-switching within realistic scenarios, students develop confidence in navigating Hong Kong's bilingual environment, which is crucial for successful veterinary practice.

By incorporating these components, the proposed curriculum aims to equip veterinary students with a comprehensive skillset, ensuring they are well-prepared to communicate effectively and compassionately in various professional settings.

Conclusion

Effective communication is essential for veterinary practitioners in Hong Kong, where bilingualism, multiculturalism, and the clinical demands of veterinary practice converge. This chapter has underscored the specific communication skills required by veterinary students and practitioners, highlighting how linguistic and cultural factors impact client interactions, interdisciplinary collaboration, and overall patient care. Through client-centred communication, cross-disciplinary teamwork, bilingual proficiency, and multimodal training, veterinary programmes can bridge the gap between academic instruction and practical demands. By integrating these competencies into the curriculum, Hong Kong's veterinary programmes can better equip their graduates to navigate the unique communication challenges of a multilingual society, enhancing the quality of care for both clients and animals. This chapter provides a framework for understanding and developing these competencies, offering practical strategies to prepare veterinary professionals for the complexities of clinical practice in Hong Kong's diverse environment.

References

Adams, C. L., & Frankel, R. M. (2007). It may be a dog's life but the relationship with her owners is also key to her health and well being: Communication in veterinary medicine. *Veterinary Clinics: Small Animal Practice, 37*(1), 1–17.

Adams, C. L., & Kurtz, S. M. (2006). Building on existing models from human medical education to develop a communication curriculum in veterinary medicine. *Journal of Veterinary Medical Education, 33*(1), 28–37.

Adams, C. L., & Kurtz, S. (2012). Coaching and feedback: Enhancing communication teaching and learning in veterinary practice settings. *Journal of Veterinary Medical Education, 39*(3), 217–228.

Almendros, A., Steagall, P. V., Lun, S. C., Speelman, J., & Giuliano, A. (2024). Challenges of the Calgary–Cambridge Consultation Guide in veterinary multicultural and multilingual scenarios and the role of veterinary translators. *Animals, 14*(15), 2270.

Bard, A. M., Main, D. C., Haase, A. M., Whay, H. R., Roe, E. J., & Reyher, K. K. (2017). The future of veterinary communication: Partnership or persuasion? A qualitative investigation of veterinary communication in the pursuit of client behaviour change. *PLoS One, 12*(3), e0171380.

Berrian, A. M., Feyes, E., Hsiao, C. Y., & Wittum, T. E. (2021). Multimodal integration of active learning in the veterinary classroom. *Journal of Veterinary Medical Education, 48*(5), 533–537.

Bonvicini, K., & Keller, V. F. (2006). Academic faculty development: The art and practice of effective communication in veterinary medicine. *Journal of Veterinary Medical Education, 33*(1), 50–57.

Coe, J. B., Adams, C. L., & Bonnett, B. N. (2008). A focus group study of veterinarians' and pet owners' perceptions of veterinarian-client communication in companion animal practice. *Journal of the American Veterinary Medical Association, 233*(7), 1072–1080.

Currie, G., & White, L. (2012). Inter-professional barriers and knowledge brokering in an organizational context: The case of healthcare. *Organization Studies, 33*(10), 1333–1361.

Dawson, S. E. (2010). Compassionate communication: Working with grief. In *Handbook of Veterinary Communication Skills* (pp. 62–99).

Englar, R. E., Williams, M., & Weingand, K. (2016). Applicability of the Calgary–Cambridge guide to dog and cat owners for teaching veterinary clinical communications. *Journal of Veterinary Medical Education, 43*(2), 143–169.

Han, L., Lee, Y., Lee, H., Lee, H., & Lee, J. I. (2024). Overcoming challenges in interdisciplinary collaboration between human and veterinary medicine. *Veterinary Sciences, 11*(11), 518.

Kogan, L. R., Accornero, V. H., Gelb, E., & Slater, M. R. (2021). Community veterinary medicine programs: Pet owners' perceptions and experiences. *Frontiers in Veterinary Science, 8*, 678595.

Li, W. (2018). Translanguaging as a practical theory of language. *Applied Linguistics, 39*(1), 9–30.

McCracken, B. J. (2016). *End-of-Life Communication in Veterinary Medicine* (Doctoral dissertation, State University of New York at Buffalo).

Morris, P. (2012). Managing pet owners' guilt and grief in veterinary euthanasia encounters. *Journal of Contemporary Ethnography, 41*(3), 337–365.

Pun, J. (2020). An integrated review of the role of communication in veterinary clinical practice. *BMC Veterinary Research, 16*(394), 1–14.

Pun, J. (2021). Comparing veterinary students' and practitioners' perceptions of communication in a bilingual context. *Veterinary Record, 189*(12), 1–11.

Pun, J. (2023). *The Role of Language in Eastern and Western Health Communication*. Routledge.

Pun, J., & Onder-Ozdemir, N. (2023). Exploring students' perceptions in sustainable disciplinary language learning in an English-medium instruction university: A case study of Hong Kong veterinary medical students. *Sustainability, 15*(2), 1279.

Scalese, R. J., & Issenberg, S. B. (2005). Effective use of simulations for the teaching and acquisition of veterinary professional and clinical skills. *Journal of Veterinary Medical Education, 32*(4), 461–467.

Shaw, J. R., & Coe, J. B. (2024). *Developing Communication Skills for Veterinary Practice*. Wiley.

Shaw, J. R., & Lagoni, L. (2007). End-of-life communication in veterinary medicine: Delivering bad news and euthanasia decision making. *Veterinary Clinics: Small Animal Practice, 37*(1), 95–108.

11

Conclusion

This concluding chapter synthesizes the core themes discussed throughout this book—*Exploring and Teaching Healthcare Communication: Clinicians' Perspectives in Hong Kong*. The book has highlighted the importance of culturally responsive communication strategies in clinical contexts, especially within Hong Kong's unique multicultural environment where Western medical practices intersect with deeply rooted Chinese cultural values. A recurring theme across the chapters is the role of family-centred decision-making, indirect communication, and holistic health approaches inherent in Traditional Chinese Medicine (TCM) as integral to effective clinician-patient relationships.

This book advocates for an integrated communication model that merges Western frameworks, such as the SPIKES and Calgary-Cambridge models, with culturally attuned practices better suited to Hong Kong's high-context, family-centred healthcare culture (Pun et al., 2018). Additionally, it examines the ethical considerations that arise in healthcare communication research, such as navigating family dominance in decision-making, obtaining informed consent, and handling sensitive data in visual documentation. By promoting culturally enriched communication practices, this chapter underscores the need for continued

J. Pun, *Exploring and Teaching Healthcare Communication*,
https://doi.org/10.1007/978-3-031-08675-5_11

adaptation of Western communication frameworks to foster trust and empathy within Hong Kong's diverse patient population.

Building on these foundational insights, the following section provides a detailed summary of the key themes explored in each chapter, illustrating how different facets of healthcare communication intersect within Hong Kong's unique cultural and medical landscape. Each chapter highlights the adaptability required of clinicians who must navigate a healthcare environment shaped by both Western medical models and traditional Chinese cultural values. From medical education to end-of-life care, Traditional Chinese Medicine, and veterinary practice, the following sections reveal how family involvement, indirect communication, and holistic approaches are interwoven into clinical practices.

Key Issues from Previous Chapters

In Hong Kong, healthcare communication is uniquely shaped by a convergence of Western medical practices and deeply rooted Chinese cultural values, making the process of patient-provider interaction more complex than in purely Western or Eastern settings. Traditional Western communication frameworks, widely used in medical training and practice worldwide, often prioritize direct, individual-centred communication, supporting patients' autonomy and personal agency in decision-making. However, these models can be challenging to apply directly in Hong Kong, where cultural expectations emphasize family-centred decision-making, respect for authority, and high-context communication. This culturally hybrid healthcare landscape demands a nuanced approach to clinical communication, one that respects traditional values while facilitating clear and compassionate interactions.

Hong Kong clinicians and healthcare educators, working within this multicultural framework, face the task of adapting established communication models to better fit the local cultural context. Areas such as end-of-life care, Traditional Chinese Medicine (TCM), and even veterinary practice are deeply influenced by these cultural considerations, underscoring the importance of context-sensitive strategies for effective clinician-patient relationships. As the following sections will demonstrate, key adaptations in medical education, EOL communication, TCM practices, and veterinary care reveal the intricate ways that family involvement, indirect communication styles, and holistic approaches are woven into the fabric of Hong Kong's healthcare environment, requiring a thoughtful integration of Western models with culturally attuned practices. In light of these cultural and contextual factors, the following sections delve into specific domains within Hong Kong's healthcare landscape, highlighting how these themes underscore the need for healthcare professionals to adopt a hybrid approach that aligns with Hong Kong's cultural dynamics, enhancing patient care through culturally attuned communication strategies.

Medical Education and Western Communication Models

The clinical communication models widely taught in medical education, such as SPIKES for delivering bad news and the Calgary-Cambridge guides for structuring consultations, provide structured and effective frameworks for patient interactions. However, these Western models often lack adaptability to Hong Kong's unique healthcare context, where family involvement and respect for authority profoundly shape the communication dynamic. Unlike the individual-centred approach commonly expected in Western settings, clinicians in Hong Kong frequently engage in more paternalistic interactions. Family members typically assume active roles in decision-making processes, reflecting the collective nature of Chinese cultural values. This dynamic requires clinicians to adapt Western frameworks by incorporating elements that acknowledge family influence while retaining patient-centred principles. Given these challenges, culturally sensitive adaptations to these models are essential for more effective communication in Hong Kong's healthcare environment, where balancing respect for authority and family involvement with patient autonomy is key.

End-of-Life Communication

Conversations surrounding end-of-life (EOL) care are especially sensitive in Hong Kong due to deeply rooted cultural taboos around discussing death directly. Chinese cultural norms often encourage family members to shield patients from distressing news to preserve emotional well-being, which can sometimes limit the patient's autonomy in making EOL decisions. This chapter examines the delicate balance clinicians must strike between respecting patient autonomy and the family's protective role during EOL discussions. Clinicians are often required to navigate these interactions with subtlety, employing indirect communication styles to align with cultural expectations while still ensuring patients are informed about their options. By sensitively integrating respect for family roles with a commitment to transparency, healthcare providers can foster EOL care that is both compassionate and culturally congruent.

Traditional Chinese Medicine (TCM) Communication

In the field of Traditional Chinese Medicine (TCM), communication is grounded in a holistic approach that aligns with Chinese philosophies of health, which view well-being as an equilibrium of the body, mind, and spirit. This holistic perspective contrasts sharply with Western medicine's more symptom-focused, direct approach. TCM practitioners in Hong Kong often employ high-context, relationship-centred communication styles that are indirect and emphasize rapport-building. This chapter explores how TCM practitioners integrate insights into patients' emotional and lifestyle factors, not just physical symptoms, to address health issues comprehensively. The practitioner-patient relationship in TCM extends beyond immediate treatment, encouraging long-term engagement that supports sustained well-being. By maintaining a high-context and culturally sensitive approach, TCM communication respects patients' individual needs within a culturally meaningful framework, ultimately enhancing patient satisfaction and therapeutic outcomes.

Veterinary Communication

Veterinary medicine in Hong Kong faces unique communication challenges due to the city's multilingual environment, where veterinarians often engage with clients in both English and Cantonese. Effective communication in this field mirrors the client-centred approach in human healthcare, requiring veterinarians to convey complex medical information clearly and empathetically. This chapter discusses the essential role of empathy, rapport-building, and adaptability in client interactions, which are central to fostering trust and understanding between veterinarians and pet owners. Bilingual communication skills are particularly important, as they ensure that both English- and Cantonese-speaking clients receive clear and compassionate information about their pets' health. By embracing a client-centred communication approach that resonates with Hong Kong's diverse cultural and linguistic landscape, veterinarians can enhance client satisfaction and improve the overall quality of care for animals.

Navigating Cultural Dynamics in Clinical Communication

The themes across these chapters underscore the complex cultural dynamics clinicians face in Hong Kong, where family involvement, indirect communication, and holistic approaches are integral to effective patient care. Clinicians are frequently tasked with balancing traditional Western communication frameworks with the specific cultural expectations of Hong Kong's healthcare environment. These cultural nuances require a hybrid communication model that integrates family-centred decision-making, indirect and contextually sensitive language, and an appreciation for holistic well-being, especially within TCM and EOL contexts. By adapting communication practices to reflect these culturally specific needs, healthcare providers can cultivate more empathetic, effective, and culturally congruent patient relationships in Hong Kong's evolving medical landscape.

Having established the foundational themes of culturally responsive communication within Hong Kong's healthcare environment, it is essential to examine the specific strategies that enable clinicians to navigate these cultural dynamics effectively. The following section outlines culturally specific adaptations that clinicians can employ to foster meaningful, empathetic relationships with patients. These strategies address the need for family-centred decision-making, indirect communication, linguistic flexibility, and holistic approaches, all of which reflect the unique cultural expectations within Hong Kong's healthcare landscape. By integrating these culturally attuned practices, clinicians can better align their communication with patients' values and expectations, thereby enhancing trust and improving health outcomes.

Cultural Adaptations in Communication Strategies

In Hong Kong's healthcare environment, effective communication requires sensitivity to the distinct cultural expectations that shape patient interactions. Unlike Western healthcare systems, which emphasize individual autonomy and direct communication, Hong Kong's context places a high value on family involvement, respect for authority, and indirect communication. These cultural nuances add layers of complexity to the provider-patient relationship, necessitating adaptations in both language and approach.

To navigate these dynamics successfully, healthcare providers must integrate culturally responsive strategies that acknowledge family roles, communicate with sensitivity around delicate topics, and adjust language use according to patient comfort and comprehension. This approach is especially relevant in settings such as end-of-life care, Traditional Chinese Medicine (TCM), and bilingual clinical interactions, where understanding and respecting cultural values can greatly enhance patient outcomes. The following sections present key adaptations in communication strategies, illustrating how these tailored approaches facilitate effective and empathetic interactions across Hong Kong's diverse healthcare landscape.

Family-Centred Decision-Making in the Communication Process

In Chinese culture, family plays a central role in healthcare decisions, often influencing or even taking on the decision-making responsibilities traditionally reserved for the patient in Western contexts. This family-centred approach is deeply rooted in the values of collectivism and filial piety, where family members' involvement is seen as a way of supporting and protecting the patient. In Hong Kong, this dynamic requires clinicians to adapt the Western model, which emphasizes individual autonomy, to acknowledge and integrate the family's voice without overshadowing the patient's wishes. Clinicians are thus encouraged to navigate this balance thoughtfully, fostering an environment where family members feel included and respected while still empowering the patient to participate actively in their healthcare decisions. This strategy requires a delicate approach to ensure that family involvement enhances, rather than diminishes, patient-centred care.

Indirect Communication

High-context communication is a common characteristic of Chinese culture, where indirect language, non-verbal cues, and euphemisms are often used, particularly when discussing sensitive subjects like terminal illness or prognosis. Rather than openly discussing difficult topics, patients and families may prefer subtle hints or indirect references, avoiding direct confrontation with distressing news. For clinicians working in Hong Kong, developing an awareness of these cultural communication norms is crucial. By recognizing and responding to patients' unspoken concerns and reading between the lines, clinicians can build rapport and provide care that aligns with cultural preferences. Training in these subtle, indirect communication strategies helps clinicians to respect cultural taboos, foster trust, and address patients' emotional needs more effectively, especially in end-of-life scenarios.

Linguistic Flexibility

The bilingual healthcare environment in Hong Kong requires clinicians to be adept at linguistic flexibility, as they often navigate between English and Cantonese. This linguistic adaptability is essential for ensuring that medical information is communicated with both accuracy and empathy. Many clinicians are trained in English, using technical terms during diagnosis and treatment planning, yet patients may feel more comfortable discussing their health in Cantonese. Clinicians must therefore be skilled in "translanguaging"—switching fluidly between languages—to convey complex medical concepts in a patient-friendly manner. By being mindful of language use and ensuring that terminology does not alienate patients, clinicians can maintain rapport and make healthcare interactions more accessible and reassuring for patients.

Holistic Approaches

Traditional Chinese Medicine (TCM) emphasizes a holistic approach that considers the patient's physical, emotional, and spiritual well-being as interconnected components of health. TCM practitioners focus on achieving balance and long-term wellness rather than merely treating isolated symptoms, which aligns with Chinese philosophical views on health. For Western-trained clinicians, incorporating some aspects of this holistic approach can significantly enhance patient care, especially in a culturally diverse setting like Hong Kong. By integrating practices that address the whole person, such as considering emotional and lifestyle factors in treatment planning, clinicians can better meet the expectations of patients who value this holistic perspective. This culturally attuned approach can deepen patient trust, improve health outcomes, and ultimately provide a more comprehensive healthcare experience that aligns with the TCM philosophy of well-being.

In addition to adapting communication strategies to fit Hong Kong's cultural context, healthcare practitioners and researchers must also navigate significant ethical considerations that arise when conducting studies and engaging with patients in this setting. The family-centred decision-making, indirect communication styles, and holistic approaches discussed in the preceding sections present unique challenges in ensuring informed consent, respecting patient autonomy, and safeguarding confidentiality. This section will explore these ethical dimensions in detail, highlighting how clinicians and researchers can uphold ethical standards while honouring the cultural dynamics that shape healthcare interactions in Hong Kong.

Ethical Considerations in Healthcare Communication Research

Informed Consent and Family Dynamics

In the context of healthcare communication research in Hong Kong, obtaining informed consent is often complicated by the central role families play in healthcare decision-making. Chinese cultural norms emphasize collectivism, where family members frequently take an active part in healthcare choices to provide support and guidance. This dynamic can inadvertently challenge a patient's individual autonomy, as family members may feel responsible for making decisions on behalf of the patient, particularly in cases involving serious diagnoses or end-of-life care. For researchers, this requires a culturally sensitive approach to the consent process, ensuring that patients are fully informed and retain their right to make decisions independently. At the same time, researchers must acknowledge the family's role, potentially involving family members in discussions to respect cultural values without compromising the patient's autonomy.

Audio/Video Recording in Clinical Settings

The use of audio or video recordings in clinical research raises significant privacy concerns in Hong Kong, especially when the topic is sensitive or emotional, such as discussions about terminal illness. Patients and their families may perceive recording as intrusive or inappropriate, fearing that their privacy will be compromised during these intimate moments. Researchers must approach this issue with care, obtaining explicit consent and explaining the purpose and handling of recordings in detail. It is also essential to address any cultural sensitivities around recording to avoid making participants uncomfortable or anxious. By maintaining transparency and emphasizing privacy protection measures, researchers can help patients and families feel more at ease with the recording process.

Confidentiality and Data Security

Given the active role that family members play in healthcare decisions, confidentiality is a particularly critical concern in healthcare communication research in Hong Kong. The close involvement of family can create situations where sensitive patient information is unintentionally shared, potentially compromising patient privacy. Researchers must take extra precautions to anonymize and securely store patient data, ensuring that identifying information is kept confidential and only accessible to authorized personnel. Developing clear protocols for data handling and communication can help prevent breaches of confidentiality, protecting patient privacy while allowing families to stay involved in a way that respects cultural norms.

Cultural Sensitivity in Research Design

Designing research methodologies that respect cultural taboos is essential when studying healthcare communication in Hong Kong. Chinese cultural norms often discourage direct discussions of death or terminal illness, and patients and families may prefer indirect language or euphemisms to handle such topics. Researchers should adopt culturally sensitive methods, such as indirect questioning, to obtain necessary information without causing distress or discomfort to participants. By respecting these cultural preferences, researchers can gather meaningful data while maintaining trust and rapport with participants, ultimately fostering a respectful and productive research environment that honours cultural values.

The ethical complexities surrounding healthcare communication research in Hong Kong highlight the need for a sensitive, culturally informed approach. By carefully navigating issues of informed consent, privacy during recordings, confidentiality, and respect for cultural taboos, researchers can maintain both ethical rigor and cultural respect in their work. These considerations underscore the importance of adapting research practices to honour patient and family dynamics, ultimately supporting more compassionate and effective healthcare communication. With these ethical foundations established, we can now turn to a broader reflection on how integrating cultural awareness into clinical practices benefits healthcare providers, patients, and the evolving healthcare landscape in Hong Kong.

Concluding Remarks

Building upon the key themes explored in this book, the concluding chapter reiterates the importance of developing culturally responsive communication strategies that are integral to healthcare practices in Hong Kong's hybrid medical environment. Drawing from interdisciplinary perspectives, this book has highlighted the significance of integrating Western frameworks, such as the SPIKES protocol and Calgary-Cambridge model, with culturally sensitive approaches that resonate with the values and expectations of Chinese patients and families. This synthesis underscores the need for clinicians to cultivate intercultural communicative competence, addressing linguistic, cultural, and relational dimensions to provide patient-centred care.

The discussions across chapters illustrate the profound influence of cultural dynamics, including family-centred decision-making, indirect communication styles, and holistic health approaches, on various domains of healthcare. In the context of critical care, the emphasis on fostering a speak-up culture among clinicians demonstrates how communication openness can mitigate risks and improve patient outcomes. For end-of-life communication, the complexities of balancing patient autonomy with familial involvement highlight the nuanced role of cultural sensitivity in enhancing trust and therapeutic alignment. Similarly, Traditional Chinese Medicine (TCM) communication exemplifies the potential of holistic, patient-centred practices to bridge traditional values and modern medical standards.

The book also sheds light on the challenges and adaptations required in multilingual healthcare settings, particularly in high-pressure environments like Accident and Emergency Departments and Intensive Care Units. The exploration of translanguaging practices and the need for standardized communication protocols reflect the intricate interplay between language, culture, and clinical efficacy. Moreover, the chapters dedicated to medical education emphasize the transformative role of culturally attuned training programmes in preparing future clinicians to navigate Hong Kong's diverse healthcare landscape effectively.

In veterinary medicine, the focus on empathy and client-centred communication mirrors the broader themes of trust-building and shared decision-making, reaffirming the universality of effective communication across medical disciplines. These insights extend the relevance of this book beyond human healthcare, advocating for a cross-disciplinary understanding of communication practices.

By integrating insights from linguistics, cultural studies, and clinical practice, this book provides a comprehensive framework for improving healthcare communication in Hong Kong and similar multicultural contexts. It calls for continued research and training initiatives that bridge the gap between Western and Chinese medical paradigms, fostering a healthcare system that is both inclusive and effective. Future endeavours should build on these foundations, exploring innovative strategies to enhance clinician-patient interactions and addressing emerging challenges in the ever-evolving landscape of global healthcare. In doing so, Hong Kong's healthcare system can serve as a model for integrating cultural competence into medical communication, offering valuable lessons for practitioners and educators worldwide.

Summary

This chapter has synthesized the essential cultural considerations in healthcare communication within Hong Kong, emphasizing how adapting Western communication models to local norms can enhance patient outcomes. Clinicians who integrate cultural awareness, linguistic adaptability, and an understanding of family-centred decision-making into their communication practices are better equipped to meet the needs of Hong Kong's diverse patient population. The integration of Traditional Chinese Medicine (TCM) perspectives further highlights the importance of holistic, patient-centred approaches, demonstrating that culturally responsive communication is crucial for building trust and ensuring effective clinical interactions.

Beyond clinical practice, healthcare communication research in Hong Kong presents unique ethical challenges. Issues related to informed consent, data privacy, and confidentiality are often complicated by family dynamics, traditional decision-making structures, and sociocultural expectations. Researchers must continue developing culturally appropriate methodologies that uphold ethical standards while respecting patients' autonomy, familial involvement, and cultural preferences. Ensuring ethical rigor in multilingual, high-context healthcare settings will be essential for advancing communication research in Hong Kong and similar environments.

While this book has provided valuable insights into culturally sensitive healthcare communication, several critical research gaps remain. Future studies should explore the long-term impact of culturally adaptive communication models, as there is limited empirical research on how hybrid approaches—blending Western models with Chinese cultural values—affect patient satisfaction, treatment adherence, and health outcomes over time. Longitudinal studies are needed to assess the effectiveness of culturally attuned frameworks in real-world clinical settings.

Another area of interest is the role of digital technology in healthcare communication. The increasing use of AI-driven translation tools, telemedicine, and digital health platforms raises important questions about their ability to bridge language gaps, improve clinician-patient interactions, and support multilingual communication. However, research must also address concerns related to accuracy, patient accessibility, and ethical implications of these technologies.

Further investigation is also needed in underexplored medical fields such as mental health, rehabilitation, and palliative care. While existing research has focused largely on oncology, emergency medicine, and TCM, disciplines like mental health communication remain underexamined in Hong Kong. Cultural stigmas often prevent open discussions about psychiatric conditions, making it essential to explore how communication strategies can be adapted to foster more supportive and effective mental healthcare.

Another significant shift in healthcare communication relates to changing family dynamics in medical decision-making. While family-centred decision-making remains a dominant cultural norm, generational shifts, increasing patient autonomy, and evolving healthcare policies are transforming clinician-patient-family interactions. Future research should examine how younger generations, changing legal frameworks, and patient advocacy movements are reshaping the traditional role of families in medical decisions.

Finally, enhancing communication training in medical education remains a key area for development. Although communication training is increasingly recognized as an essential component of medical and nursing education, there is limited research on the effectiveness of structured training programmes that incorporate cultural competence, interdisciplinary collaboration, and real-world simulations. Evaluating how different training approaches influence clinical communication skills will be crucial for shaping future curricula and ensuring that healthcare professionals are prepared to navigate culturally diverse patient interactions.

As Hong Kong's healthcare landscape continues to evolve, the integration of culturally responsive communication practices will be essential for clinicians, researchers, and policymakers. The development of hybrid frameworks that respect both Western medical principles and Chinese cultural traditions will help shape a more inclusive, patient-centred, and ethically sound healthcare system. By addressing these research gaps and embracing interdisciplinary, technology-driven, and ethically conscious approaches, Hong Kong has the potential to serve as a global model for culturally informed healthcare communication in increasingly multicultural societies.

References

Pun, J., Chan, E. A., Wang, W., & Slade, D. (2018). Health professional–patient communication practices in East Asia: An integrative review of an emerging field of research and practice in Hong Kong, South Korea, Japan, Taiwan and Mainland China. *Patient Education and Counseling, 101*(7), 1195–1206. https://doi.org/10.1016/j.pec.2018.01.019

Index

J. Pun, *Exploring and Teaching Healthcare Communication*,
https://doi.org/10.1007/978-3-031-08675-5

T

U

V

The manufacturer's authorised representative in the EU is Springer Nature Customer Service Centre GmbH, Europaplatz 3, 69115 Heidelberg, Germany. If you have any concerns regarding our products, please contact ProductSafety@springernature.com

Printed and bound by CPI Group (UK) Ltd, Croydon, CR0 4YY
30/09/2026
02225595-0003